FISH OIL

The Natural
ANTI-INFLAMMATORY

JOSEPH C. MAROON, M.D., and JEFFREY BOST, P.A.C.

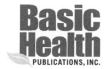

Basic
Health
PUBLICATIONS, INC.

The information contained in this book is based upon the research and personal and professional experiences of the authors. It is not intended as a substitute for consulting with your physician or other healthcare provider. Any attempt to diagnose and treat an illness should be done under the direction of a healthcare professional.

The publisher does not advocate the use of any particular healthcare protocol but believes the information in this book should be available to the public. The publisher and authors are not responsible for any adverse effects or consequences resulting from the use of the suggestions, preparations, or procedures discussed in this book. Should the reader have any questions concerning the appropriateness of any procedures or preparation mentioned, the authors and the publisher strongly suggest consulting a professional healthcare advisor.

Basic Health Publications, Inc.
28812 Top of the World Drive
Laguna Beach, CA 92651
949-715-7327 • www.basichealthpub.com

Library of Congress Cataloging-in-Publication Data

Maroon, Joseph C.
    Fish oil : the natural anti-inflammatory / Joseph C. Maroon and Jeff Bost.
      p. cm.
    Includes bibliographical references and index.
    ISBN-13: 978-1-59120-182-3
    ISBN-10: 1-59120-182-9
  1. Inflammation—Alternative treatment. 2. Fish oils—Therapeutic use.
I. Bost, Jeff. II. Title.

    RB131.M37   2006
    616'.0473—dc22

                             2006005353

In-house Editor: Nancy Ringer
Typesetting and Book design: Gary A. Rosenberg
Cover Design: Mike Stromberg

Printed in the United States of America

10   9   8   7   6   5   4   3   2

Contents

Introduction, 1

1. Understanding Inflammation and Chronic Disease, 5

2. Drugs: Helpful or Harmful?, 18

3. Omega-3 Essential Fatty Acids: The Natural Anti-Inflammatories, 33

4. Fish Oil: An Omega-3 Powerhouse, 48

5. Fish Oil at Work: Clinical Trials, 58

▶ *Vascular Disease, 58*

▶ *Stroke, 76*

▶ *Diabetes, 78*

▶ *Rheumatoid Arthritis, 80*

▶ *Spine Pain, 82*

▶ *Osteoarthritis, 82*

▶ *Inflammatory Bowel Disease, 83*

▶ *Systemic Lupus Erythematosus, 84*

▶ *Multiple Sclerosis, 85*

▶ *Asthma, 86*

▶ *Dry Eye Syndrome, 88*

▶ *Macular Degeneration, 89*

▶ *Eczema, 90*

▶ *Psoriasis, 90*

▶ *Pregnancy and Infancy, 91*

▶ *Postpartum Depression, 92*

▶ *Menstrual Pain, 92*

▶ *Attention-Deficit Hyperactivity Disorder, 93*

▶ *Developmental Coordination Disorder, 95*

▶ *Autism and Asperger's Syndrome, 95*

▶ *Alzheimer's Disease, 96*

▶ *Parkinson's Disease, 99*

▶ *Depression, 99*

▶ *Bipolar Disorder, 101*

▶ *Schizophrenia, 101*

▶ *Cancer Protection, 102*

6. Fish Oil Supplements: Finding a Good-Quality Product and the Appropriate Dosage, 107

Glossary, 121

References, 125

Index, 167

About the Authors, 170

Introduction

Anyone who's ever sprained an ankle, slammed a finger in a door, had an ear infection, or met any other kind of physical misfortune—in other words, just about every member of the human race—has seen firsthand the effects of inflammation: heat, swelling, redness, pain, and/or loss of function. Inflammation in these circumstances is a normal physiological reaction, and it is just one of many of the body's self-protective mechanisms.

But the news on inflammation is not all good. Although it helps the body protect and heal itself, over the long term inflammation can produce chronic pain, breakdown of cartilage and muscle, and increased blood clotting, and it may cause genetic changes leading to various cancers. In fact, recent medical research now confirms that the root cause of many chronic diseases, ranging from arthritis, heart disease, and cancer to attention-deficit hyperactivity disorder, asthma, eczema, and depression, is inflammation.

Should we draw a link between the prevalence of these diseases in Western society and the state of inflammation in the general population? The answer is a resounding "Yes!" For years health experts have fingered poor diet and sedentary lifestyle as the culprits behind the growing state of poor health in the American public. In this book we unveil a third and most dangerous villain: chronic inflammation, a silent and insidious condition that is the root cause and common factor with poor diet and inactivity leading to most of the chronic diseases that rob us of our health and lives.

Pharmaceutical companies have spent billions of dollars in an attempt to understand the biochemistry of inflammation. They have found that interfering with one specific chemical enzyme, known as cyclooxygenase (COX), can greatly reduce inflammation from many causes. In fact, in 2003 the amount of money spent in the United States for COX inhibitors, more commonly called nonsteroidal anti-inflammatories (NSAIDs), such as ibuprofen, aspirin, steroids, Aleve, Bextra, Vioxx, and Celebrex, added up to approximately $20 billion. Unfortunately, studies showed that many of these pharmaceutical COX inhibitors can greatly increase the risk of stomach irritation, ulcer, and potentially lethal gastric hemorrhage—not the sort of side effects most people are comfortable risking! A class of selective COX-2 inhibitors developed in the late 1990s was designed to prevent these stomach problems. By 2002 these selective COX-2 inhibitors accounted for 51 percent of all COX inhibitors used in the United States. The drugs' developers believed that these COX-2 inhibitors would allow users to either stop or dramatically reduce their concomitant use of drugs to protect their stomachs. But a 2004 study found that patients taking these COX-2 drugs were actually even more likely to be taking stomach-protective drugs. Finally, in September 2004, due to several studies showing an increased risk of heart attack and stroke in those who used it, the COX-2 inhibitor Vioxx, one of the most popular prescription drugs ever, was pulled from the market. Bextra followed, and now Celebrex, another selective COX-2 inhibitor, is under rigorous review.

What does all this have to do with fish oil? We see the ravages of inflammation on a daily basis in our patients with spinal arthritis, disc herniation, and brain and spinal cord trauma. We have witnessed catastrophic complications and even deaths that were caused by commonly used pharmacological agents to reduce pain and inflammation, so we began to search for alternatives. Based on epidemiological and clinical research, and backed up by our own experiences, we have come to believe that the omega-3 essential fatty acids found in fish oil are the most under-recognized and also the most potent natural anti-inflammatories available—and they do not have the potentially lethal side effects of pharmacological agents.

We initially began recommending therapeutic doses of fish oil to patients with spinal pain from herniated discs or degenerative arthritis. We found that over 60 percent of them, in a few weeks, could stop taking their prescribed pharmacological anti-inflammatory while maintaining a steady pain-reduction and anti-inflammatory response. As team neurosurgeon for the Pittsburgh Steelers, Dr. Maroon recommended fish oil to elite athletes for inflammatory conditions such as joint pain, overuse injuries, and exercise-induced asthma. The response was also positive. Indeed, we have had indisputable and overwhelming positive response to the use of fish oil as an anti-inflammatory for quite some time now. And because most people—including physicians—are unaware of the prevalence of chronic inflammation and the potency of fish oil as an anti-inflammatory, we feel that it is imperative to spread the good word.

The remainder of this book delves into the biochemistry of inflammation. We have done our best to render the discussion suitable for all readers—no advanced degrees required! At the same time, we have strived to make the discussion comprehensive, so that our readers will come away with a good understanding of the ways in which chronic inflammation plagues our society and an appreciation for the finer virtues of fish oil's omega-3 fatty acids. In short, the discussion could be summarized, chapter by chapter, as follows:

1. Inflammation is normally a protective physiological mechanism, but many factors common in Western society can cause it to become a long-term condition, with dire consequences.

2. Pharmacological anti-inflammatory drugs are effective in reducing inflammation but have potentially lethal side effects, rendering them impractical for use on a long-term basis.

3. Omega-3 essential fatty acids may be at least as effective as pharmacological anti-inflammatories, and they are much safer.

4. Fish oil is the best source of these omega-3 essential fatty acids.

5. Hundreds of clinical trials support the efficacy of fish oil's omega-3 essential fatty acids in preventing, mitigating, and remedying an incredible range of health conditions.

6. All fish oil is not the same. Finding a high-quality pure and potent product is imperative, as is taking the appropriate amount.

If the content of the book can be summarized in these six points, why bother reading on? Because the exploration of fish oil's uses and mechanisms of action is a truly fascinating one, offering intriguing insights into the biochemistry of health and exciting prospects for the treatment and prevention of some of our most feared ailments, from cancer and stroke to Alzheimer's, autism, and depression. Best of all, it offers a glimpse of the bright future Western medicine can hope to have as it learns to welcome and work with the great array of powerful, potent healing remedies the natural world has to offer. With over 14 percent of the United States' annual gross national product being spent on health care, we must understand what that healthcare system has to offer us, and what it lacks. By continuing to support and promote only traditional (expensive) medical techniques, we may be neglecting a very powerful natural ally that has the potential to rebalance our body and return us to good health.

CHAPTER 1

Understanding Inflammation and Chronic Disease

To understand how and why fish oil is such an effective anti-inflammatory, we must first understand how inflammation works and why this process exists. The inflammatory process is a natural response of the body to an injury, whether it is of physical, chemical, or infectious origin. In most cases inflammation is a protective response and is a prelude to healing.

Despite the fact that inflammation is inherently a protective mechanism, its effect on our tissues and organs may be excessive, may cause permanent or temporary damage, and above all almost always involves pain. Control of excessive inflammation, therefore, is key to our health and well-being.

THE IMMUNE SYSTEM RESPONSE

The immune system is designed to protect the body, and especially to provide a physical barrier to foreign invaders. Cells in the skin are considered to be part of the immune system, as are tears and nasal mucus, which contain natural chemicals that digest bacteria and their toxins. When attacked, our immune system reacts in two protective ways. The first response is based on innate immunity, or inborn defenses that employ a team of specialized immune-system cells. Some time later, a process called acquired immunity kicks in, when our immune system "learns" about various problems and designs a specific response to target each kind. Acquired immunity involves the production of antibodies and certain specialized immune cells that are tailored to destroy microbes or other foreign substances.

Many different types of cells fight on our immune system's front line, with each type performing a unique and necessary role. In doing so, immune cells carry ammunition: chemicals and proteins that work to kill bacteria and disable viruses. These chemicals and proteins are part of the body's inflammatory response to any transgression, be it bacterial, viral, traumatic, or autoimmune.

CLASSIC INFLAMMATION

The human body has evolved over the millennia into a formidable force of complex and effective defense mechanisms that we are still trying to understand. Our primitive ancestors were able to survive and thrive without the knowledge or benefit of good hygiene, sterile dressings, and antibiotics. That survival ability comes not only from conscious decisions (for example, to avoid or run from danger) but also from what our body does automatically on a daily basis to defend itself against injury, mutated/damaged cells, and invasion by foreign substances and disease.

Skin, the first line of defense, is a barrier to pathogens. Other barriers include our mucous membranes, body secretions (tears, perspiration, and saliva), and some reflexes like coughing and sneezing. If an irritant gets past these defenses (or arises from within the body), our white blood cells engulf and destroy it. Our bodies also have specialized natural killer cells, called T cells, that can recognize when a cell membrane becomes abnormal (as would be the case for a cancerous cell) and kill it. The process by which the body reacts to an irritant and tries to get rid of it (or at least limit its harmful effects) is called inflammation. Without this automatic defense mechanism, we would have little hope for survival in our hostile world.

The inflammatory response is often very rapid, such as occurs after a bee sting. It is not controlled by any brain or organ function. Instead, all the immediate reactions arise from the cells, and more specifically the cell membranes, that have been damaged. The speed of the response often can save us from further injury, as the pain alerts us to the danger as, for example, when we run from the beehive.

The classic signs of inflammation are heat, swelling, redness, pain, and loss of function. Heat and redness are the result of increased blood supply due to reflex dilation of the smaller arteries in the affected area. Chemical mediators act on the cells lining the small blood vessels (capillaries and venules) at the site of injury to make them more permeable; as a result, blood plasma leaks from the small blood vessels into surrounding tissues, causing swelling. Pain and loss of function are associated with chemical mediators released by damaged tissues that act on local nerve endings, as well as the increased pressure on nerve endings caused by swelling in the area.

The release of chemical mediators in the affected area starts a cycle of further increase in the permeability of the blood vessels, leading to more swelling, heat, redness, and pain. Next, blood cells migrate into the tissues; either they arrive through these same blood vessels or they are preexisting in the area, as sentries that stand always at the ready to defend against attack and release various chemical mediators. One of these mediators is histamine, which comes from

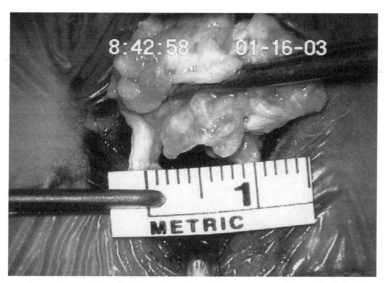

Figure 1.1. An inflamed herniated disc. The inflammatory response caused by the disc material results in pain, swelling, and eventual loss of nerve function, since the inflamed disc can release cytokines and other inflammatory factors that irritate the surrounding tissues and nerve fibers.

mast cells and other leukocytes (white blood cells). This phase of inflammation is often referred to as being "histamine dependent," and it is the reason antihistamines work in the early phases of inflammation.

A second wave of the inflammatory process soon follows and is characterized by the release of specialized molecules called kinins, complement, and prostaglandins. These substances are formed or released from damaged blood and tissue cell membranes. They cause further damage and increase the inflammatory response. The inflammatory reaction continues for as long as the noxious agents persist. When the noxious agents are contained or eliminated, they are removed by the lymphatics (that is, the lymph glands, which can become swollen), and metabolized by enzyme systems.

Thus, the inflammatory response can be thought of as a defensive battle. The body is like a fortified fortress with its many defensive systems on standby and poised to repel an attack. The attack comes without notice and may originate anywhere inside or outside the body. The instantaneous reaction is both to allow a massive response to flood the area and to send out the alarm that this area is under attack and needs help. Waves and waves of additional helpers then come to complete the job and mop up the injured areas. Only at this point may the affected person recognize the problem and take some measures to avoid further injury and to tend to the ailment.

THE COMPLEMENT SYSTEM

The complement system consists of a host of molecules that reside in our blood in an inactive form. Complement molecules spring to action when they sense bacteria, injury, or other immune-system triggers. When activated, complement proteins cause a range of responses associated with initiating and maintaining inflammation. These include changes in blood vessel walls (making them more permeable, or leaky), the summoning of various types of immune cells, and the production of other substances that promote inflammation. A molecule called C-reactive protein (CRP) interacts with the complement system. The presence of CRP in blood is a telltale sign of inflammation because it is normally not present in appreciable amounts in the blood of healthy people. It is a biological marker that may warn of a potential heart attack risk before any symptoms are noticed.

Two major players in the inflammatory battle are the white blood cells (leukocytes) and the eicosanoids; we'll discuss them in greater detail next.

LEUKOCYTES

Leukocytes, also known as white blood cells, are the most active specialized cells during an inflammatory reaction. In contrast to red blood cells, whose singular role is to carry oxygen to all the organs, white blood cells have many and varied roles. The several types of leukocytes include neutrophils, monocytes, macrophages, eosinophils, lymphocytes, basophils, and mast cells. All of these cells originate as stem cells inside bone marrow. This marrow can be very responsive to the body's defensive needs and can rapidly produce additional white blood cells if the body is under attack. (In the face of a severe attack the marrow can release some white blood cells that are not completely mature yet. Detection of these immature cells in the body can signal a severe infection.) Each type of white blood cell has a specialized function to fight an outside invasion and are by far the most active cells in the body to prevent disease. They can initiate and continue the inflammatory response, when needed, in every part of the body. They are truly the main infantry of our bodies' defenses.

EICOSANOIDS: THE "GOOD" AND THE "BAD"

We are all familiar with the hormones released by various glands in the body such as the pituitary, the thyroid, and the adrenal. Much less recognized or understood are the eicosanoids, which are hormonelike substances produced in all of the 60 trillion cells in our body. They fall into three main categories—

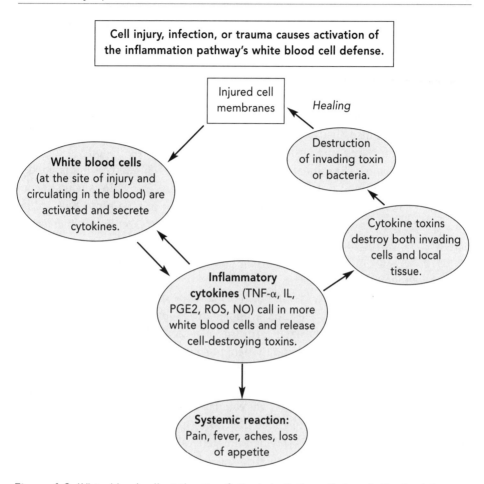

Figure 1.2. White blood cells at the site of attack, both those that are in the local tissue (macrophages) and those that are bloodborne (neutrophils, lymphocytes, monocytes, and basophils), jointly initiate the inflammatory response by releasing cytokines to call in more white blood cells. Cytokines also release toxic substances that can destroy both invading cells and local tissue. Cytokines have been found to be a major cause of the systemic symptoms of pain, fever, and aches that sometimes accompany the inflammatory response.

prostaglandins (PG), leukotrienes (LT), and thromboxanes (TX)—along with several minor categories.

Like hormones, eicosanoids are chemical messengers that play a role in every function of the human body. Unlike hormones, however, they are destroyed by local enzymes within seconds or minutes of formation. This limits their activities to the area in which they are released.

Having the capacity to produce chemical messengers at an immediate cellular level allows the body to produce quick, localized action in almost any tissue or organ. The most general need for rapid, local action is in the response to trauma. Therefore, eicosanoids are most often concerned with clotting, inflammation, and the initiation of immune defense.

Although eicosanoids are essential for life and perform many "good" functions such as preventing blood clots, reducing pain, and enhancing the immune system, there are also "bad" eicosanoids that enhance blood clotting, cause pain, and suppress the immune system. A balance between the "good" and "bad" effects of eicosanoids is critical for health; for example, blood clotting is good if we are injured but bad if it occurs in a coronary artery, and pain is usually considered negative but can be lifesaving if it enables us to take protective action. As we shall see, however, consequences of excessive production of "bad" eicosanoids include the most common chronic diseases and the most frequent causes of morbidity and mortality: cancer, heart disease, stroke, arthritis, depression, and Alzheimer's disease.

The membrane of every cell in our body is made up of phospholipids, which consist of two fatty acid molecules, a phosphate group, an alcohol, and a glycerol. Eicosanoids are synthesized from the fatty acids in these phospholipids. Because the fatty acids are constantly being used up, they must be replaced frequently. Those replacements come in the form of essential fatty acids (EFAs). These fatty acids are "essential" because the body does not synthesize them and we must take them in via the food we eat. There are two kinds: omega-3 EFAs, which are generally considered "good" because they produce anti-inflammatory eicosanoids, and omega-6 EFAs, which are generally considered "bad" because they produce inflammatory eicosanoids. The distinction between the "3" and the "6" is a biochemical one relating to the position of double bonds in the fatty-acid molecule. The most important and most bioactive of the omega-3 EFAs are eicos-

Table 1.1. The "Good" and "Bad" Effects of Eicosanoids Summarized	
"Good" Eicosanoids (derived from omega-3 EFAs)	**"Bad" Eicosanoids** (derived from omega-6 EFAs)
Prevent blood clots caused by platelet aggregation	Promote blood clots caused by platelet aggregation
Cause vasodilatation of blood vessels	Cause vasoconstriction of blood vessels
Reduce pain	Promote pain
Decrease cell division	Promote cell division
Enhance the immune system	Depress the immune system
Improve brain function	Depress brain function

EICOSANOID TERMINOLOGY

Eicosanoids can be grouped into various "families" or series. There are, for example, three series of prostaglandins and thromboxanes: one derived from dihomo-gamma-linolenic acid, a derivative of arachidonic acid (series 1); one derived from arachidonic acid itself (series 2); and one derived from EPA (series 3). Eicosanoids in the same family tend to have, in general, similar effects. Each eicosanoid is referred to by a letter, followed by the number of the series it belongs to: for example, prostaglandin I_2, thromboxane A_2, or leukotriene A_4.

apentaenoic acid (EPA) and docosahexaenoic acid (DHA), which are found in abundance in fish oil. The most common omega-6 EFA is arachidonic acid (AA).

Conversion of phospholipid essential fatty acids to various eicosanoids is affected by various enzymes released from the cell membrane, with two of the most important of these being cyclooxygenase (COX) and lipoxygenase (LOX). Knowing how these enzymes work is critical to understanding why many of today's modern drugs and supplements are effective at relieving inflammation and pain. Both cyclooxygenase and lipoxygenase are used by the body's cells to change the essential fatty acids EPA and DHA, which are found within the cell membranes, into very potent anti-inflammatory eicosanoids. These same enzymes, however, can also convert AA in the cell membranes into inflammatory eicosanoids that are almost always associated with pain, swelling, and dis-

Table 1.2. The Effects of Eicosanoids on Metabolic Function			
Organ System	**Effects of Eicosanoids**	**EPA and DHA Source**	**AA Source**
Blood Vessel	vasoconstriction		X
	vasodilation	X	
	permeability		X
Platelets	adhesion, aggregation		X
	antiaggregation	X	
Lung	bronchial constriction		X
	bronchial dilation	X	
Stomach	acid secretion		X
	peristalsis		X
Tissue	pain		X

ability. The omega-3 and omega-6 lines of essential fatty acids are therefore said to "compete" for these enzymes; when omega-6 EFAs, for example, exist in overwhelming proportion to omega-3 EFAs, they may use up an overwhelming proportion of the available cycloogygenase and lipoxygenase. The discovery of this enzymatic process has led to the development of the most popular line of pharmaceutical drugs ever created, the nonsteroidal anti-inflammatory drugs (NSAIDs), which block COX enzymes and therefore block the inflammation pathway. (For more detail about the actions of these important essential fatty acids, see Chapter 3.)

Prostaglandins

Prostaglandins are the target of most treatments to stop or slow the inflammatory process. These eicosanoids not only are synthesized when tissues are injured but are found in every cell in the body—and we have 60 trillion cells! They play a critical role as local messengers in all normal body functions. Once produced, prostaglandins do not persist long at their site of formation. Instead, they are released at the local site and are rapidly metabolized and absorbed. Most prostaglandins are metabolized so rapidly that they do not reach the blood circulation system for redistribution.

Prostaglandins and Pain

High concentrations of prostaglandins cause pain by direct action upon nerve endings. More typically, however, they are found at low concentrations and markedly increase sensitivity to pain. The pain threshold may be so altered that even normally painless stimuli may be painful. This effect of prostaglandins is long-lasting and cumulative, so that continued production of just small amounts of prostaglandins can sensitize nerves to irritants. The increased sensitivity to pain can manifest not only locally (such as at the site of previous trauma that hurts long after it appears to have healed) but also centrally, since prostaglandins can sensitize nerve receptors in the central nervous system (the brain and spine).

Prostaglandins and Inflammation

There are many contributors to the inflammatory process, and prostaglandins are among the more significant ones. As chemical messengers they can stimulate increased blood flow, chemotaxis (movement of various cells, particularly leukocytes), subsequent dysfunction of tissues and organs, and, as we discussed, pain. The phagocytes (macrophages and monocytes that employ phagocytosis, or the engulfing of bacteria or any toxic substance in the area of injury) summoned by prostaglandins use enzymes to digest foreign materials. These enzymes may be discharged or may leak from these cells into the body's tissues, stimulating the production of more prostaglandins and thus setting up a cycle in which reinforcements of these specialized white blood cells are called in, which rapidly increases the inflammatory response.

As long as the noxious agent or tissue injury that caused the initial inflammation persists, prostaglandins will continue to be produced and will add to the inflammatory process.

This low-level inflammation persisting in the body is now thought to be one of the main causes of many chronic diseases, such as heart disease, Alzheimer's disease, autoimmune diseases, arthritis, and even diabetes. Since we live in a society with so many environmental and foodborne irritants that can spark the inflammatory response, these diseases may just be the "natural" end result.

Prostaglandins and Pyrexia (Fever)

During an inflammatory response, infectious agents, toxins, and tissue fluids can enter the body's circulation system. As a result, in acute cases prostaglandins are produced in the central nervous system, specifically the anterior hypothalamus (the temperature-regulating part of the brain), resulting in fever. With fever, depressed energy (malaise) and loss of appetite may occur.

The fever produced by prostaglandins can be countered with anti-inflammatory agents that inhibit prostaglandin production. In the classic inflammatory response, both pain and fever are the first signs of inflammation to be relieved by anti-prostaglandin therapy. Swelling and redness are alleviated more slowly.

Positive Roles of Prostaglandins

Although prostaglandins are implicated in chronic inflammation, they can play both positive and negative roles in the body and therefore should not be thought of as just "the bad guys." Prostaglandins play a significant role as local messengers in many normal physiological functions, including the following:

- Prostaglandins are involved in maintaining normal function of the cardiovascular, pulmonary, renal, and gastrointestinal systems.

- Prostaglandins can stabilize blood pressure.

- In the lungs prostaglandins not only modify pulmonary circulation but also modify ventilation by constricting or contracting airways.

- In the newborn, as soon as the lungs are functional, prostaglandins redirect umbilical blood flow and divert venous blood to the lungs for proper aeration.

- In the gastrointestinal tract, prostaglandins decrease the secretion of gastric juice and increase the secretion of intestinal mucus. They increase the fluid content of the gut and may increase gut motility.

Anti-inflammatory pharmaceuticals that alter or block prostaglandin function affect not only the "bad" effects (inflammation, pain, fever) but also the "good" effects (balanced optimal blood pressure and air flow to the lungs, balanced gastric pH, maintenance of intestinal mucus function and renal function). For example, some anti-inflammatory drugs that block prostaglandin production prevent the formation of both the prostaglandin responsible for inflammation and the prostaglandin used by the body to protect the stomach from stomach acids. The result is reduced inflammation but also gastrointestinal ulcer. In fact, every year 100,000 people experience bleeding ulcers as a result of the use of anti-inflammatories such as ibuprofen (Motrin, Advil), Aleve, and Vioxx.

Leukotrienes

Leukotrienes play a major role in the inflammatory response to injury. They are potent inflammation activators. Leukotrienes are formed via the lipoxygenase enzyme from the breakdown of arachidonic acid. Recently released drugs used to treat asthma work by blocking the lipoxygenase enzyme. The leukotriene LTB_4 and cysteinyl leukotrienes are potent chemotactic agents that, during an asthma attack, can attract pro-inflammatory white blood cells, such as neutrophils and eosinophils, into lung tissue. Within the airways and vascular smooth muscle of the lungs they can stimulate mucus secretion by increasing microvascular permeability. Besides asthma, leukotrienes have been implicated in many inflammatory diseases, such as psoriasis, rheumatoid arthritis, and inflammatory bowel disease.

Thromboxanes

Thromboxanes have a powerful action on the airways. In asthmatics thromboxanes are responsible for small airway constriction (by inducing contraction of smooth muscles in the airways), and they increase congestion by increasing mucus secretion.

Eicosanoids and Diet

Omega-6 EFAs are found in high concentrations in red meat, grains, some vegetable seed oils, and the many products made therefrom. Omega-6 EFAs can be converted into the pro-inflammatory eicosanoids, of which arachidonic acid is the most common. Omega-3 EFAs are found primarily in fish oil, and to a much lesser extent in flaxseed, walnuts, and green plants. Omega-3 EFAs can be converted into anti-inflammatory eicosanoids.

The pro-inflammatory eicosanoids produced from the omega-6 pathway have what are generally considered negative effects. For example, prostaglandin E_2 causes an increase in leakage through the blood vessels, elevation in temperature, and increased sensitivity to pain. Leukotriene A_4 causes spasm of the small airways, difficulty breathing, and increased mucus secretion. Thromboxane A_2 causes clumping of platelets and constriction of blood vessels and airways.

Countering these reactions are the positive effects of the eicosanoids produced from the anti-inflammatory omega-3 pathway. Prostaglandin E_3, for example, decreases swelling, reduces sensitivity to pain, and lessens the recruitment of inflammatory white blood cells, and leukotriene A_5 dilates the airways and decreases mucus secretion.

Our diet of either more or less omega-3 or omega-6, therefore, plays a critical role in affecting the equilibrium essential for regulating eicosanoid production and hence our health. A diet rich in the omega-6 EFAs from red meat, grains, and vegetable seed oil products will tend to drive the cellular production of eicosanoids toward the pro-inflammatory path. In contrast, a diet rich in omega-3 EFAs from fish and/or fish oil supplements will drive the cellular production of eicosanoids toward the anti-inflammatory path. As we shall see in Chapter 3, an imbalanced diet weighted toward omega-6 EFAs, at the expense of omega-3 EFAs, can result in chronic systemic inflammation, which in turn can lead to a host of serious health conditions.

SYSTEMIC INFLAMMATION

So far, we have described the local inflammatory response at the site of injury, trauma, or infection. If, however, local inflammation cannot be controlled or the immune system is overwhelmed, the inflammatory response may involve systemic (body-wide) changes. These systemic changes can be acute and can lead to shock or even death. Systemic changes in inflammation are mediated by cytokines, which are proteins produced by white blood cells, mostly macrophages, that act as chemical messengers and can act on other cells. Interleukin-1 (IL-1) is a cytokine that can travel through the blood to affect endothelial cells (the lining of blood vessels) throughout the body. Tumor necrosis factor-alpha (TNF-α), also a cytokine, can work in a similar way. These two proteins can travel far from the original site of trauma by way of the bloodstream to produce many serious symptoms.

Fever results when IL-1 travels to the anterior hypothalamus, the temperature-regulating center in the brain. There, it stimulates cells to release arachidonic acid, which is converted into prostaglandins by cyclooxygenase. These prostaglandins reset the body's thermostat to a higher temperature. The body reacts as though it is too cold—muscles shake to generate heat, and the flow of blood to the skin is decreased. This continues until the new higher temperature setting (a fever state) is reached. Aspirin and other anti-inflammatories reduce fever by inactivating cyclooxygenase and preventing the formation of these prostaglandins.

IL-1 also stimulates the release of bone marrow's stored reserves of mature neutrophils. Once these have been exhausted, the body sends out immature neutrophils until the cytokines stop calling for more.

Cytokines also stimulate the rapid transformation of the arachidonic acid in the membranes of skeletal muscle cells into inflammatory prostaglandins that cause the release of amino acids into the blood, thereby breaking down muscle and causing the aches and pains associated with injury or infection.

In response to the production of inflammatory cytokines, red blood cells may "clump" or aggregate, at a rate proportional to the degree of inflammation. Because of this tendency to clump, a simple blood test, called the "sed rate" test, can be used to determine the level of inflammation in the body. This test measures the erythrocyte sedimentation rate, or the rate at which red blood cells clump in response to circulating cytokines. The clumped red blood cells can be seen as sediment at the bottom of a tube of blood. The faster the blood settles, the greater the amount of inflammation.

CHRONIC INFLAMMATION

Clearly, our success as a species is dependent on our immune and inflammatory response systems. However, inflammation is a double-edged sword, because it can be beneficial or detrimental, depending on the circumstances. The major benefit of inflammation is to summon the body's defensive mechanisms to fend off any outside invaders and to begin the repair and healing process following an injury. When inflammation becomes a chronic state, however, devastating consequences may occur in the form of cancer, heart disease, stroke, and arthritis, to name a few.

Chronic cellular inflammation can occur if the cause of the inflammation is continually reintroduced or if the acute inflammatory response is not able to eliminate it. Such a state is not uncommon in today's society, since we are exposed to incredible amounts of toxins on a daily basis. Some of these toxins we bring upon ourselves, such as from poor food choices, smoking, and sun exposure. Some arise from things we can't control, like our genetics, exposure to pollution, or accidents and trauma. Chronic cellular inflammation is more likely to occur if the eicosanoid production pathway favors pro-inflammatory factors over anti-inflammatory ones on a persistent, systemic basis. As we shall discuss in Chapter 3, the Western diet has seriously compromised the balance of eicosanoid synthesis in the body, to the detriment of our well-being.

As acute inflammation turns into a chronic situation, short-lived neutrophils are replaced by longer-lived macrophages and lymphocytes. These cells may cause destruction of tissue even while that tissue is trying to heal. During this phase an excessive amount of blood vessels and scar tissue can form. This process is often made worse by the way the inflammatory process tries to wall off or contain the injured area. Macrophages will consume the source of irritation, but in doing so either they will become immobile and stay in that area to eventually form a mass or they will rupture. In the case of atherosclerosis or heart disease, that rupture can cause an acute heart attack; in the brain, it can cause a stroke.

Chronic inflammation can also be *silent:* a low-grade, destructive inflammatory response that occurs without the classic overt signs of inflammation, such as pain, heat, and redness. This condition is, we believe, commonplace in the Western population and a major contributor to development of fatigue, obesity, chronic pain, and general poor health, as well as the onset of a wide range of diseases.

Prevention of chronic inflammation, therefore, becomes imperative. Pharmacological treatment was once thought to be the answer to this problem, but as we'll see in the next chapter, its serious and potentially lethal side effects far outweigh its benefits.

CHAPTER 2

Drugs: Helpful or Harmful?

A s we discussed in Chapter 1, inflammation is one of the major causes of many chronic diseases. Heart disease, heart attack, stroke, and clot formation all can be linked to a prolonged state of excessive inflammation in our blood vessels. Complications of diabetes, Alzheimer's, obesity, and autoimmune disorders such as arthritis and lupus are related to cellular inflammation and its harmful effects. Though the medical establishment has long known of these and other health conditions, we have failed to recognize chronic inflammation as the common link among them.

Nevertheless, pharmaceutical companies have developed many medications that help reduce inflammation and thereby help relieve the symptoms and reverse the progress of inflammation-related conditions. As with any pharmacological product line, the industry giants have invested huge sums in developing the latest, most effective, "safest" anti-inflammation drugs—and for the most part have failed, unable to come up with a product that doesn't have very serious side effects. In this chapter, starting with aspirin and leading up to the most recent COX-2 inhibitors (such as Vioxx, Bextra, and Celebrex), we will review how these drugs—each one of them once lauded as the greatest discovery ever— can have very ugly and potentially life-threatening side effects.

UNDERSTANDING THE RISKS OF MEDICATIONS

Unfortunately, oftentimes the best-intended treatments, especially pharmaceutical drugs, have serious unintended side effects that are discovered only after injuries or even deaths have occurred. The recognition of these problems is often delayed by many reasons, beginning with the approval process for a new drug.

FDA Approval and Its Limitations

The U.S. Food and Drug Administration (FDA) was established in 1906 with the passage of the Federal Food and Drugs Act and now has a staff more than 9,000 employees and an annual budget of $1.3 billion. Within the FDA, the Center for Drug Evaluation and Research (CDER) was developed to assure the safety and effectiveness of drugs that are available to the American people. The process by which a pharmaceutical company develops and seeks CDER approval of a new drug may take years and can cost billions of dollars, without any assurance that the drug will ever be approved. The major part of this process is human safety and efficiency trials to determine not only the drug's effectiveness but also any risks or side effects. The general time frame for these trials is one to two years. Approximately one to two thousand subjects are followed and monitored during a trial's duration. If the results of these trials show the drug to be successful, the pharmaceutical company then presents these results to CDER for approval. If it grants approval, CDER will set down specific indications for use, dosage guide-lines, and precautions for the drug as based on the clinical trials, along with doc-umentation of any side effects noted during the trial.

Once approved, the new drug is made available to physicians to prescribe to those patients they believe may benefit from it. Now several interesting things can occur. First, despite the specific recommendations and precautions that accompany this new drug, a physician has the right to prescribe the drug to any patient he or she thinks appropriate (in medical jargon, this is called "off-label use"). This means that patients who may not have the same disease or condition as those who participated in the original trials may be exposed to the effects of the drug. Additionally, as the drug is now exposed to a larger population than it was in the original clinical trial population, and usually for a longer period of time, the potential exists for recipients to develop different and potentially more serious complications. Also, although the drug may have been proven effective for only one condition, new studies may be developed to evaluate the drug for different indications. Aspirin is a classic example, as it is now used as both an anti-inflammatory pain reliever as well as a preventive medication for stroke and heart attack.

Weighing Risks versus Benefits

The medical community is fortunately populated not only with persons who want to invent new medical treatments and drugs but also with those who are skeptical of "wonder drugs" or treatments that seem too good to be true or have not been rigorously studied. One of the major responsibilities of the scientific and medical communities is to communicate new findings and report potential problems and side effects, traditionally through publication in scientific journals. More recently, researchers have begun going directly to the general public through the media to report problems in cases where they feel the situation is critical.

In 1998, J. Lazarou, B. H. Pomeranz, and P. N. Corey published the results of a meta-analysis of the incidence of adverse drug reactions (ADRs) that had resulted in either hospitalization or death in the United States in 1994. They found that annually 2,216,000 people were hospitalized due to ADRs, and 106,000 of these had fatal ADRs, making these reactions the fifth leading cause of death. In 2004, J. Pirmohamed and colleagues looked at almost 20,000 patients admitted to two British hospitals over a six-month period and found that 1,225 admissions, or 6.5 percent, were related to ADRs, and of those, 28 patients died. The drugs most commonly causing these admissions included low-dose nonsteroidal anti-inflammatory drugs (NSAIDs). The most common reaction was gastrointestinal bleeding, which was also was the most common cause of death. And in just these two hospitals the annualized cost to care for these ADRs was projected to be almost $1 billion.

In the United States the estimated cost per patient per hospitalization to care for an ADR from an NSAID is $15,000 to $20,000; the annual expenditure for treatment of NSAID-related gastrointestinal complications exceeds $2 billion. In 2001, M. Langman found that 40 percent of all admissions for peptic ulcer in those patients older than sixty years and 40 percent of the deaths attributed to peptic ulcers were related to the use of NSAIDs. Factors such as advanced age, a history of ulcers, alcohol use, and the combination of aspirin and NSAIDs can all make the risk of side effects from these prescription and nonprescription anti-inflammatories much higher.

So why do the pharmaceutical industry and medical community continue to manufacture and prescribe NSAIDs when they are known to be potentially dangerous? The fact is that these drugs as a class tend to be very effective at reducing inflammation and pain, and additionally they replace what is thought to be even more potentially dangerous but also very effective anti-inflammatory drugs: steroids.

The use of steroids as powerful anti-inflammatories is well described. Corticosteroid medications are synthetic versions of natural hormones (cortisone and hydrocortisone) produced by the body's adrenal glands. Both natural and synthetic corticosteroids have powerful anti-inflammatory effects; they reduce the increased blood flow and migration of leukocytes seen in inflammation and decrease the production and action of the complement proteins, prostaglandins, cytokines, and thromboxanes that induce inflammation. But they also have well-described side effects related primarily to a decrease in the body's healing capabilities, including a decrease in the normal protective aspects of the inflammatory response, and also have significant bone (osteoporosis) and gastric side effects (ulcers and intestinal bleeding). The potential severity of these complications generally limits steroids to short-term use or for use in very serious conditions such as severe lung disease when the alternative to these medications may be death.

So NSAIDs are safer than steroids. But they themselves are not considered generally safe. In fact, as we'll show later in this chapter, even the newest COX-2-inhibiting NSAIDs still carry the very side effect they were designed to eliminate: gastric complications, including potentially lethal gastric hemorrhage. Is there a better alternative? For sure. We'll start talking about it in the next chapter. But before we get there, we need to break down the reasons why NSAIDs have these serious side effects. We'll start by looking at the original NSAID: aspirin.

ASPIRIN: THE ORIGINAL NSAID

The use of aspirin, or salicylic acid, marked the beginning of pharmaceutical treatment of inflammation and pain. This very complex chemical can be found in its natural state in the bark of the willow tree. It was used by Hippocrates, the father of medicine, and there is evidence that it has been used as a natural anti-inflammatory and pain reliever for thousands of years. Only relatively recently, on March 6, 1889, was it patented in its synthetic form by the Bayer Pharmaceutical Company.

In the 1960s researchers found that aspirin blocks the enzyme cyclooxygenase-1 (COX-1) from being used to synthesize the eicosanoid thromboxane A_2 in platelets. This eicosanoid causes platelet aggregation (sticking together of platelets), vasoconstriction (narrowing of blood vessels), and vascular proliferation (increased formation of blood vessels), all of which can lead to heart attack or stroke. The blockage is permanent for the lifespan of the platelets, which is about nine days; in other words, the antiplatelet effect persists until newly formed platelets have been released. Aspirin can also block some production of prostacyclin (PGI_2), found within blood vessel walls, which normally prevents platelets from sticking to the blood vessel lining (endothelium). This effect, however, is only temporary, and therefore the overall positive effect of aspirin as an NSAID lies in its ability to reduce platelet function and clotting.

Clinical Uses of Aspirin

In 1998 the FDA updated the labeling requirements for aspirin, allowing manufacturers to claim that aspirin could reduce the risk of the following medical problems:

- Stroke—in those who have had a previous stroke or a transient ischemic attack (a mini-stroke, possibly a warning of a stroke to come)

- Heart attack—in those who have had a previous heart attack or who experience angina (chest pain); aspirin reduces the risk of death or complications from a heart attack if it is taken at the first sign of a heart attack

• Recurrent blockage of arteries—for those who have had heart bypass surgery or another procedure to clear blocked arteries, such as balloon angioplasty or carotid endarterectomy

Under this ruling, the recommended dose for cardiovascular use is 50 to 325 milligrams (mg) once daily, or 75 to 325 mg in cases of angina and previous heart attack. Diabetics are often considered an at-risk population for vascular clotting and the higher dosage of aspirin is generally recommended for them.

Complications

The use of aspirin in the prevention of cardiovascular disease is now well established; an estimated 50 million Americans have started taking aspirin for this purpose over the past two decades. However, aspirin can cause serious bleeding complications. The risk of gastrointestinal bleeding, for example, is significantly increased by long-term aspirin use. And the same quality that gives aspirin its potential benefit—its ability to inhibit clotting of the blood—may increase the risk of excessive bleeding, including the possibility of bleeding in the brain. Many newer studies show that even the lower doses now recommended for vascular protection may not completely reduce this bleeding risk.

> **CAUTION**
>
> Combining aspirin with other NSAIDs can lead to serious bleeding complications and even death and is not recommended.

Some other possible risks are:

• **Stomach irritation.** Aspirin is acidic and can irritate the stomach lining and cause heartburn, pain, nausea, vomiting, and, over time, more serious consequences such as internal bleeding, ulcers, and holes in the stomach or intestines. Additionally, it can block the production of PGI_2 (prostacyclin), which is protective to the stomach lining. Some studies now show that up to 17 percent of all hospital admissions for bleeding peptic ulcers are due to aspirin use. Chronic alcohol users (three or more alcoholic beverages a day) may be at increased risk of stomach bleeding and liver damage from aspirin use.

• **Ringing in the ears.** At high doses, aspirin may cause temporary ringing in the ears and hearing loss, which usually disappear when the dose is lowered.

• **Allergy.** Facial swelling and sometimes an asthma attack may occur in the 2 out of every 1,000 people who are allergic to aspirin.

- **Reye's syndrome.** Aspirin should not be used to treat children's flulike symptoms or chicken pox because of the risk of this rare but serious disease.

Because of its risks, aspirin is not approved for decreasing the risk of heart attack in healthy individuals. Despite its many known benefits, aspirin should not be taken for its cardiovascular benefits except after consultation with a qualified healthcare provider who can evaluate the benefits versus the risks of long-term use for individual cases.

MODERN NSAIDS: TARGETING COX

In contrast to aspirin, the new classes of NSAIDs were developed specifically to target COX. In 1971, Sir John Vane, who subsequently won a Nobel Prize for his work, suggested that inhibition of prostaglandin pro-inflammatory factors could be achieved through blockage of the COX enzyme, and a variety of NSAIDs were developed to achieve that blockage. Vane's prediction turned out to be correct: blocking the COX enzyme results in less prostaglandin E_2, a pro-inflammatory cytokine, and therefore less inflammatory response and less pain.

This new class was heralded as a miracle drug, and within several years an estimated 15 to 20 million people were using NSAIDs on a long-term basis in the United States. NSAIDs are now among the most commonly used pharmaceutical agents in the United States. Over 70 million NSAID prescriptions are written each year, and 30 billion over-the-counter NSAID tablets are sold annually. Some investigators have estimated usage at 5 to 10 percent of the adult American population, and among the elderly—a group at higher risk of NSAID-induced gastrointestinal complications—the prevalence of NSAID use is as high as 15 percent.

From Nonselective to Selective

In the late 1980s and early 1990s, it was discovered that COX exists in the body in one of two forms, labeled COX-1 and COX-2. The class of NSAIDs that had just been developed was nonselective, meaning that the drugs blocked both COX-1 and COX-2. Although these NSAIDs had been shown to have substantial anti-inflammatory and pain-relieving effects, they also have serious gastric side effects, including gastrointestinal bleeding requiring hospitalization and even leading to death. The holy grail of NSAID research became the development of a potent anti-inflammatory pain reliever without the annoying and potentially lethal gastric side effects. Researchers believed that the answer lay in selective NSAIDs, which would block just COX-2, reducing inflammation and thereby pain, while preserving COX-1's protective gastric function. With this new group of COX-2-specific inhibitors, which includes Celebrex, Bextra, and Vioxx, researchers thought they had found the perfect anti-inflammatory.

Nonselective NSAIDs

Nonselective NSAIDs reduce inflammation because they block COX-2, which is responsible for the production of inflammatory prostaglandins, but they also cause gastrointestinal mucosal injury because they block COX-1, which is responsible for the production of prostaglandins that protect the gastric mucosa (stomach lining).

Protection of the gastric mucosa from the effects of gastric juices is a complex process, but in essence it is managed by four distinct operators that all must work together: the mucous layer, epithelial bicarbonate (a natural antacid), cellular repair mechanisms, and mucosal blood flow. All of these factors are dependent in part on local production of prostaglandins. When COX-1 is blocked, fewer protective prostaglandins are produced, which disrupts the mucous layer and decreases the secretion of epithelial bicarbonate, which can lead to the buildup of hydrogen ions (acids) and cause further damage to the mucosa. This injury is made worse by the reduced ability of the mucosa to repair itself and the decline in mucosal blood flow. The result is the typical gastrointestinal mucosal injury seen with NSAID use.

Selective NSAIDs

While COX-1 is responsible for prostaglandins that protect the gastric mucosa, COX-2 produces inflammation factors in the body that are responsible for inflammation-induced pain. Thus it is the inhibition of COX-2 that is responsible for the anti-inflammatory and pain-relieving effects of NSAIDs. COX-2-specific inhibitors (such as Vioxx, Bextra, and Celebrex) selectively block the activity of COX-2 only, resulting in analgesia (pain relief) and anti-inflammatory effects without the adverse gastrointestinal results that result from blockage of COX-1.

Many of the original nonselective NSAIDs, such as naproxen, were supplanted by this newer COX-2-selective group because of the perceived gastro-protective effect. It was thought that a major side effect of these drugs had been overcome and we again could have our safe and effective "miracle" drug for pain relief. Unfortunately, this stance has been proven to be somewhat optimistic, since many newer studies indicate some risks of gastric irritation with the COX-2-selective NSAIDs as well, but generally the side effects do not occur with the same severity as with the nonselective NSAIDs.

NSAID Side Effects

Gastrointestinal side effects associated with NSAID use are common. NSAID-associated indigestion occurs in up to 50 percent of patients who use these drugs, and heartburn, nausea, vomiting, and abdominal pain can also be ob-

CAUTION

Do not take NSAIDs if you:

- Are pregnant or trying to become pregnant (acetaminophen may be safer)
- Are breast-feeding (acetaminophen may be safer)
- Have a peptic ulcer
- Have a history of stomach ulcers or gastrointestinal bleeding
- Have nasal polyps
- Have kidney or liver disease
- Have a history of allergic reactions to aspirin or related medications
- Are anemic
- Have a blood-clotting defect
- Are taking any of the following medications: blood thinners (anticoagulants), corticosteroids (such as prednisone), lithium, or oral antidiabetic medication

served. Up to 100 percent of patients taking long-term nonselective NSAIDs will demonstrate hemorrhage or bleeding of the stomach lining, about 50 percent will have erosions (small breaks in the stomach lining), and 20 percent or more will have ulceration (injury extending through the muscular layer of the stomach lining). Oddly, those who have ulceration are more likely to be free of symptoms of heartburn and therefore at greater risk for acute stomach bleeding and perforation.

Fortunately, only 1 to 3 percent of patients develop serious gastrointestinal side effects while taking NSAIDs. The problem is that with millions of people being prescribed NSAIDs annually, even a relatively small incidence of complications has resulted in a massive number of affected persons.

Some experts have estimated that NSAID-induced gastrointestinal complications result in more than 100,000 hospitalizations and as many as 16,500 deaths, with costs exceeding $2 billion annually. The relative risk for hospitalization and death in patients who use NSAIDs has been estimated to be 2.5-fold to 5.5-fold greater and 4-fold greater, respectively, than in patients who do not use NSAIDs. It has also been estimated that one-third of the cost of arthritis care falls under management of adverse gastrointestinal effects from NSAIDs. Thus, NSAID use results in substantial morbidity, mortality, and healthcare utilization and cost.

Risk factors for gastrointestinal complications include a history of peptic ulcer disease, gastrointestinal complications, major cardiovascular disease, or rheumatoid arthritis; concomitant use of anticoagulants, corticosteroids, or stomach medications (such as cimetidine, omeprazole, or ranitidine); advanced age or generally poor health; recent initiation of NSAID therapy (within three months); and use of high doses of NSAIDs, multiple NSAIDs, or both. *Helicobacter pylori* infection involving the stomach, cigarette smoking, and alcohol consumption are possible additional risk factors for NSAID-induced ulcers.

Less common side effects include kidney or liver damage, worsening of high blood pressure and fluid retention, skin rash, and mild drowsiness. Very rarely, ibuprofen, naproxen, and rofecoxib have caused meningitis; people who have an autoimmune disease such as systemic lupus erythematosus may be more at risk for developing this complication.

Table 2.1. Nonselective NSAIDs in Order of Relative Risk of Gastric Complications
LOWEST RISK
nabutmetone (Relafen)
salsalate
etodolac (Lodine)
ibuprofen
aspirin
dicofenac (Voltaren)
sulindac (Clinoril)
diflunisal (Dolobid)
naproxen (Aleve)
indomethacin (Indocin)
tolmetin sodium (Tolectin)
fenoprofen calcium (Nalfon Pulvules)
ketoprofen (Orudis, Oruvail)
piroxicam (Feldene)
flurbiprofen (Ansaid)
meclofenamate sodium (Meclomen)
ketorolac (Toradol)
HIGHEST RISK

WHERE IT WENT DEADLY WRONG

On December 1, 1998, the FDA voted to approve celecoxib (Celebrex), the first selective COX-2 inhibitor, for treating arthritis pain. Rofecoxib (Vioxx) was approved several months later, followed by valdecoxib (Bextra).

The number of prescriptions for nonselective (COX-1 and COX-2) inhibitors such as Motrin quickly dropped as the new selective COX-2-inhibiting NSAIDs began to grow in popularity. By its seventh week on the market, Celebrex had surpassed Viagra, the impotence medication, in generating record numbers of daily prescriptions early in its marketing. The big three (Celebrex, Vioxx, and Bextra) quickly became the mainstay for treatment of chronic pain conditions related to inflammation. In the United States alone in 2003 sales of these three drugs surpassed $9 billion. The general acceptance of these drugs was due to the perception that they didn't have the serious gastrointestinal side effects that had been associated with the nonselective class of NSAIDs.

However, the dominance of this new class of COX-2 inhibitors came crashing down when on September 30, 2004, the FDA acknowledged the voluntary withdrawal from the market of Vioxx (rofecoxib), a selective COX-2-inhibiting NSAID manufactured by Merck & Co. The concern mentioned by both Merck and the FDA was the reported increased risk of serious cardiovascular events, including heart attacks and strokes, found in patients participating in a clinical trial to determine whether Vioxx could reduce the risk of colon cancer. In April 2002, well before the 2004 withdrawal, Merck had been forced to place an additional warning on Vioxx packaging that informed users of increased cardiac risks based on results of Merck's own post-approval study, but despite those findings the drug had remained on the market until September 2004.

Since then, most selective COX-2 inhibitors and even a few nonselective inhibitors have been called into question as possibly having serious vascular side effects in both the heart and the brain.

Where Is the Evidence?

The first of these damning trials, VIGOR (Vioxx Gastrointestinal Outcomes Research), was published in November 2000. This was a prospective, double-blind, random trial comparing two groups of rheumatoid arthritis patients—one group took Vioxx (50 mg daily), while the other group took naproxen (500 mg daily)—to determine the incidence of upper gastrointestinal (GI) side effects. Although Vioxx was found to have fewer GI side effects compared to naproxen, the safety data revealed that it was associated with a significant increase in myocardial infarctions (MI), unstable angina, stroke, and transient ischemic attack. The difference in cardiovascular events was due primarily to a higher incidence in nonfatal heart attacks in the Vioxx group. Based on this study the FDA required a cardiac and stroke warning label to be placed on the Vioxx bottle in April 2002.

A second Vioxx trial revealed an increased risk of cardiovascular events at an even lower dosage. The APPROVe (Adenomatous Polyp Prevention on Vioxx) trial studied the risk of recurrent colon polyps in patients with a history of this

THE VIOXX TIMELINE

May 1999—FDA approves Vioxx.

March 2000—Merck reveals that a new study found Vioxx patients had double the rate of serious cardiovascular problems as those who took naproxen.

November 2000—The *New England Journal of Medicine* publishes the VIGOR study. In the VIGOR trial, the rate of serious gastrointestinal events among those receiving Vioxx was half that of those receiving a traditional NSAID (naproxen), but a significant increase in the incidence of myocardial infarction was observed.

February 2001—An advisory panel recommends the FDA require a Vioxx label warning of the possible link to cardiovascular problems.

September 2001—The FDA warns Merck to stop misleading doctors about Vioxx's effect on the cardiovascular system.

April 2002—The FDA tells Merck to add information about cardiovascular risk to Vioxx's label.

August 2004—An FDA researcher presents results of a database analysis of 1.4 million patients; it concludes that Vioxx users are more likely to suffer a heart attack or sudden cardiac death than those taking Celebrex or a nonselective NSAID.

September 23, 2004—Merck learns the results of the Adenomatous Polyp Prevention on Vioxx (APPROVe) study, which was designed to determine the drug's effect on benign colonic tumors.

September 30, 2004—Merck withdraws Vioxx from the United States and the more than 80 other countries in which it was marketed. This action was taken because of a reported significant increase in the incidence of serious thromboembolic adverse events in the APPROVe group that received 25 mg of rofecoxib per day as compared with the placebo group. Increased blood pressure and a higher incidence of myocardial infarction and thrombotic (clot-forming) stroke was reported after a year or more of treatment. Patients taking Vioxx in this study were twice as likely to suffer a heart attack or stroke as those on placebo.

condition and whether Vioxx would reduce the reoccurrence. In September 2004, after eighteen months, and well before the actual end date of the study, the Vioxx patients were found to have twice the risk of developing an MI as compared to the placebo group, and the study was halted.

As a result of these and other studies, and also as a result of a number of vocal cardiologists calling for the ban of Vioxx, Merck voluntarily removed Vioxx from the worldwide market.

Concerns with Other NSAIDs

Since the September 2004 recall of Vioxx, many questions have arisen regarding the potential long-term side effects and health risks of selective COX-2 inhibitors and all other types of NSAIDs. As a class, COX-2 inhibitors were the most commonly prescribed drugs for the treatment of arthritis and joint pain in the world. COX-2 inhibitors were also prescribed for many forms of back and spine pain. The recall highlighted the safety concerns related to all types of NSAIDs. Other studies examining the selective COX-2 inhibitors Celebrex and Bextra as well as nonselective NSAIDs are now being intensively reviewed.

While earlier short-term studies had not clearly associated a significant cardiovascular risk with Celebrex, the APC (Adenoma Prevention with Celecoxib) trial provided conflicting information. APC evaluated whether Celebrex could prevent the development of adenomatous polyps. The cardiovascular safety data showed that death from cardiovascular causes (MI, stroke, or heart failure) was 1 percent in the placebo group, 2.3 percent in group taking 200 mg of Celebrex twice daily, and 3.4 percent in the group taking 400 mg of Celebrex twice daily. This trial was halted in December 2004, before its completion, due to concerns about the dose-related increase in cardiovascular events associated with Celebrex.

Adverse cardiovascular findings are also being investigated for Bextra. In a 2005 study at the Texas Heart Institute, N. A. Nussmeier and colleagues examined the use of Bextra to treat postoperative pain following coronary artery bypass grafting (CABG). They evaluated 1,671 patients and found significantly more blood-clotting events (in the heart, brain, and lungs) in the Bextra treatment group than in the placebo group. They concluded that "selective COX-2 inhibitors should be avoided in patients undergoing CABG," adding that this caution should probably be extended to patients undergoing vascular procedures for atherosclerotic disease, although this population has not been studied.

Explaining the Clotting Risk

These studies, primarily in the fields of cancer prevention, especially of the colon, and pain control have shown that use of selective COX-2 inhibitors

Table 2.2. Different Types of NSAIDs*	
Generic Name	**Brand Name(s)**
Salycylic Acids	
aspirin (acetylsalicylic acid)	Ascriptin, Bayer, Ecotrin
choline magnesium trisalicylate	Trilisate
diflunisal	Dolobid
salsalate	Disalcid, Salflex
Propionic Acids	
fenoprofen	Nalfon
flurbiprofen	Ansaid
ibuprofen	Advil, Motrin, Nuprin
ketoprofen	Actron, Orudis, Oruvail
naproxen	Aleve, Anaprox, Naprelan, Naprosyn
oxaprozin	Daypro
Acetic Acids	
diclofenac	Cataflam, Voltaren
indomethacin	Indocin
sulindac	Clinoril
tolmetin	Tolectin

increases the risk of vascular clotting problems, particularly among patients that are already at an increased risk of clots, such as the elderly and those with underlying vascular disease. The longer these NSAIDs (Vioxx, Bextra, and Celebrex) are used, the greater the risk is thought to be. The main risk is that over time the normal protective prostaglandin immune factors that prevent platelets from clotting and adhering to blood vessel walls (endothelium) are blocked by the inhibition of the COX-2 enzyme, thereby increasing the risk of clot formation, which can lead to stroke or heart attack. This is especially true for those who are at high risk, such as those who have had a prior heart attack or recent bypass graft or vascular stent.

Prostacyclin (PGI_2), a prostaglandin that is the predominant COX-2 product in endothelium, has many positive effects. It inhibits platelet aggregation, causes vasodilatation, and prevents the overabundance of vascular smooth-muscle cells, which can lead to plaque formation. Prostacyclin's cardiovascular protective effects balance those of thromboxane A_2, the major COX-1 product of platelets, which causes platelet aggregation, vasoconstriction, and vascular proliferation.

Generic Name	Brand Name(s)
Enolic Acids	
meloxicam	Mobic
piroxicam	Feldene, Fexicam
Fenamic Acids	
meclofenamate	Meclomen
mefenamic acid	Ponstel
Napthylalkanones	
nabumetone	Relafen
Pyranocarboxylic Acids	
etodolac	Lodine
Pyrroles	
ketorolac	Toradol
COX-2 Inhibitors	
celecoxib	Celebrex
valdecoxib	Bextra
rofecoxib	Vioxx (*recalled in 2004*)

*Includes nonselective COX inhibitors and selective COX-2 inhibitors

Traditional nonselective NSAIDs inhibit both thromboxane A_2 (derived from the COX-1 pathway) and prostacyclin (derived from the COX-2 pathway) and thus maintain the balance, whereas Vioxx and the other selective COX-2 inhibitors leave thromboxane A_2 unaffected and able to work unopposed. This predisposes patients on selective COX-2 inhibitors to a higher risk of vascular clotting, which can result in myocardial infarction (heart attack) or thrombotic stroke. A depression of just prostacyclin formation can also elevate blood pressure, accelerate atherogenesis (plaque formation), and predispose a patient to an exaggerated thrombotic response to the rupture of a vascular plaque. The higher the patient's underlying risk of cardiovascular disease, the more likely it is that such events would result in a stroke or heart attack.

WHAT HAVE WE LEARNED?

These latest events again teach us that despite the best intentions and safeguards the FDA cannot completely protect the American public from potentially serious drug-related complications. In the real world, where many patients receive many different drugs at the same time, the complex interactions between the body's metabolism and these chemicals can have many unknown consequences. We now know that most of the potential gastrointestinal benefits of the selective COX-2 inhibitors are wiped out when the patient is also on aspirin. Long-term clinical trials with large numbers of patients are very expensive, but as we have seen with the selective COX-2 inhibitors, if the studies upon which the drugs' approval was based had been continued for a year or more, most of the dangerous side effects would have been discovered before the study results were submitted to the FDA for approval. Of course, we all want safe and effective relief from inflammation and pain, but the price we've paid for pharmaceutical drugs such as steroids (immune suppression, bone loss, and increased blood sugar), nonselective COX inhibitors (gastric ulcer, bleeding, and death), and selective COX-2 inhibitors (stroke and heart attack) has been high, and we must now look for safer and more natural alternatives that may have similar positive effects and little to no side effects.

CHAPTER 3

Omega-3 Essential Fatty Acids: The Natural Anti-Inflammatories

Traditional medicine now recognizes that many diseases, both chronic and acute, as well as the aging process itself can often be linked to chronic inflammation. Based on these facts, many medical treatments and pharmacological drugs have been developed for the sole purpose of blunting or blocking the inflammatory process. Despite this huge effort in terms of time and billions of dollars spent, the current state of treatment is often ineffective and in many cases can even lead to serious complications.

Alternative research into inflammation has now shown that certain dietary supplements can reduce levels of pro-inflammatory factors, with significantly fewer side effects. The discovery of this fact has led to a dramatic shift in how we, as a practicing medical team, view not only inflammation-related diseases but also the concept of disease prevention. In our opinion, the best of these natural anti-inflammatory supplements is fish oil. We have dedicated the remaining chapters of this book to understanding the biochemical and clinical nature of this miraculous product of the sea.

The first step toward understanding how and why fish oil is such an amazing anti-inflammatory is to examine the role of its primary constituents—omega-3 essential fatty acids—in human physiology. As we'll see, an imbalance of essential fatty acids, which is primarily an omega-3 deficiency, is a major contributor to the state of chronic inflammation that NSAIDs were designed to address.

UNDERSTANDING FATTY ACIDS

In the early 1930s scientists became intrigued with the results of a study of rats on a restricted-fat diet. They found that the exclusion of fat from the diet of rats led to growth retardation, reproductive disturbances, scaly skin, kidney lesions, and excessive water consumption. Once fats were reintroduced to the rats' diet, these conditions resolved. This study led to the discovery of essential fatty acids (EFAs), or fatty acids that the body requires but cannot synthesize, and that are therefore essential for us to consume in our diet. Researchers next discovered molecules derived from these EFAs that have various biological activities. The first molecule discovered, called a prostaglandin, stimulated blood vessels and smooth muscles. Since that time, many new biologically active molecules derived from EFAs have been discovered, and as a class they are known as eicosanoids. As we discussed in Chapter 1, they fall into three major categories—prostaglandins, thromboxanes, and leukotrienes—and they play an important role in the body's inflammatory response.

To understand how the essential fatty acids found in fish oil influence our body's functions and especially the inflammatory reaction, it is important to understand the basic chemistry of fatty acids. A fatty acid molecule is a long hydrocarbon (hydrogen and carbon) chain capped by a carboxyl group. The length of the chain and the number and type of bonds it has determines the type of fatty acid it forms.

Fats generally exist as three fatty acid molecules bonded together with a glycerol molecule; this type of fat is called a triglyceride. The types of fatty acids within the triglyceride structure control many things about the fat, including whether it is solid or liquid at room temperature, how your body processes it, and how healthy it is for your body.

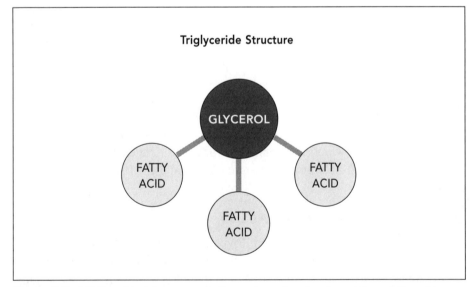

Figure 3.1. A triglyceride fat composed of one glycerol molecule and three fatty-acid molecules.

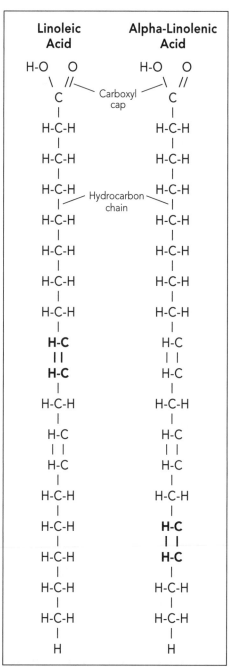

Figure 3.2. The chemical structure of linoleic acid, an omega-6 fatty acid, and the chemical structure of alpha-linolenic acid, an omega-3 fatty acid.

Saturated versus Unsaturated

Fatty acids can be grouped into two categories: those whose hydrocarbon chains are fully saturated with hydrogen atoms and those whose chains are not. Carbon atoms have only four "open" bonds available. In a fatty-acid hydrocarbon chain, at least two of those bonds connect each carbon atom to adjacent carbon atoms. When the remaining two bonds for all the carbon atoms in the chain are uniformly filled with hydrogen atoms, a fatty acid is "saturated." Fats made of saturated fatty acids are solid at room temperature.

If a carbon atom in the hydrocarbon chain is double-bonded to an adjacent carbon atom, however, leaving just one bond available for hydrogen, it is "unsaturated," because a hydrogen atom is now missing from the hydrocarbon chain. Fats made of unsaturated fatty acids are liquid at room temperature. An unsaturated fatty acid containing just one double bond is called monounsaturated. Fatty acids that have multiple double bonds are called polyunsaturated.

Altering Fat Structures

Corn oil has a high concentration of linoleic acid. Because linoleic acid is polyunsaturated, corn oil is liquid at room temperature. If you wanted to solidify it, you must subject it to high heat to break some of the double carbon bonds and add hydrogen atoms to more fully saturate the fatty acids.

The process of saturating the fatty-acid hydrocarbon chains with hydrogen is called hydrogenation, and it creates partially hydrogenated oil, which is the main ingredient in vegetable shortening and margarine. *A byproduct of this artificial saturation is trans fatty acid.*

Trans Fatty Acids

Unsaturated fatty acids have double carbon bonds that come in two forms: *trans* and *cis.* These two forms are differentiated by the direction of folding that occurs at the double bonds, which affects the location of the hydrogen atoms bonded to the double-bonded carbon atoms. Unsaturated fatty acids in their natural form are cis fatty acids, in which the folding is in the "right" direction and the hydrogen atoms are on the same side of the double bond. *This shape allows cis fatty acids to be more easily incorporated into cell membranes and allows for the membranes' fluidity and functional activities.*

Trans fatty acids are chemically identical to cis fatty acids but fold in an unnatural direction at the double bonds, so that the hydrogen atoms are on opposite sides of the double bonds. The unnatural folding results from the application of high heat, whether during the hydrogenation process or in cooking (such as in deep-fat frying).

Trans fats are found in many fried foods including french fries and fried chicken. They are also found in the

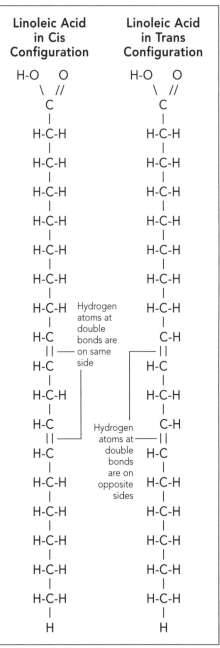

Figure 3.3. Linoleic acid in both cis and trans configuration. The chemical structure is identical in the two forms; only the configuration is different—but what a difference that makes, in terms of the health cost to our bodies!

form of partially hydrogenated oil in many packaged foods such as doughnuts, cookies, and crackers. In the United States, the fat content in a typical french fry is about 40 percent trans fatty acids, and the fat content in many popular cookies and crackers ranges from 30 to 50 percent trans fatty acids. The fats in doughnuts are about 35 to 40 percent trans fatty acids.

The process of hydrogenation was developed primarily because, in contrast to saturated and unsaturated fats, hydrogenated fats can be stored almost indefinitely and do not need to be refrigerated. That artificial stability, however, has led to a high health cost, which a whole generation is now paying for. *Trans fatty acids are now known to increase blood levels of low-density lipoprotein (LDL), or "bad" cholesterol, while lowering levels of high-density lipoprotein (HDL), or "good" cholesterol.* This is one of many factors, along with obesity, sedentary lifestyle, and poor nutrition, that have led to heart disease and stroke being the top causes for death and disability in the industrial world. A 1993 study by W. C. Willett and colleagues found that men who consume the most trans fatty acids have twice the risk of developing heart disease as those men who consume the least. Additionally, because of the unnatural folding at their double carbon bonds, trans fatty acids require the body to use extra enzymes to process them; these enzymes are then unavailable for processing the essential fatty acids that make up cell membranes.

When trans fatty acids were first developed, packaged food manufacturers were not required to list trans fat content on their products' nutrition labels, and consumers had no way of knowing how much trans fat was in the products they

Table 3.1. Dietary Fats and Their Generalized Effects on Cholesterol Levels			
Type of Fat	**Main Source**	**State at Room Temperature**	**Effect on Cholesterol**
Mono-unsaturated	Olives; olive, canola, and peanut oils; cashews, almonds, peanuts, and most other nuts; avocados	Liquid	Lowers LDL; raises HDL
Poly-unsaturated	Soybean, safflower, and cottonseed oils; fish oil	Liquid	Lowers LDL; raises HDL
Saturated	Whole milk, butter, cheese, and ice cream; red meat; chocolate; coconuts, coconut milk, and coconut oil	Solid	Raises both LDL and HDL
Trans	Most margarines; vegetable shortening; partially hydrogenated vegetable oil; deep-fried chips; many fast foods; most commercial baked goods	Solid or semisolid	Raises LDL; lowers HDL

consumed. Nevertheless, the Food and Drug Administration (FDA) advised that intake of trans fats should be as low as possible. In July 2003, after considerable pressure from consumer watchdog groups and researchers from around the world, the FDA announced a rule requiring food manufacturers, as of 2006, to list the content of trans fatty acids on nutrition labels. Since then, many major food-processing companies and restaurants have begun using safer alternatives to trans fatty acids in their products and foods. Researchers believe that *replacing partially hydrogenated fat with healthier unsaturated vegetable oils will prevent 30,000 to 100,000 premature deaths from heart disease each year in the United States.*

ESSENTIAL FATTY ACIDS AND INFLAMMATION

As discussed earlier, EFAs are fats that we must consume in our diet, since our body does not manufacture them. They are divided into two groups: omega-6 EFAs, which include linoleic acid and its derivatives, and omega-3 EFAs, which include alpha-linolenic acid and its derivatives. Both omega-3 and omega-6 EFAs are polyunsaturated. What distinguishes the two types is the placement of the first double bond in their hydrocarbon chains: the omega-3 EFAs have their first double bond located at the third carbon position, whereas the omega-6 EFAs have their first double bond at the sixth carbon (see Figure 3.2 on page 35). Although all the EFAs can be found in human food sources, only linoleic acid and alpha-linolenic acid are considered truly essential, since the body contains enzymes with which it can synthesize all the other EFAs from these two fatty acids.

Table 3.2. Major Omega-3 and Omega-6 Essential Fatty Acids	
Omega-3	**Omega-6**
alpha-linolenic acid (ALA)	linoleic acid (LA)
eicosapentaenoic acid (EPA)	arachidonic acid (AA)
docosahexaenoic acid (DHA)	gamma-linolenic acid (GLA)
	dihomo-gamma-linolenic acid (DGLA)

Essential fatty acids are necessary for the proper development and functioning of the brain and nervous system, as well as for the production of eicosanoids (thromboxanes, leukotrienes, and prostaglandins), which regulate numerous body functions including blood pressure, blood viscosity, vasoconstriction, immune response, and inflammatory response. EFAs also are critical for the growth or division of all cells and the formation of healthy cell membranes. During cell division, the cell membrane must expand so that the new cell can be completely divided from the original. EFAs are responsible for the fluidity in the cell membrane that makes possible this expansion and the sealing off of the new and original cells. The concentrations of the different types of EFAs in the phospholipid layer of cell membranes determines the particular character and function of those membranes. Cell division continues throughout our life, slows with age or disease, and stops as we die.

The cell membrane—whether it is exposed to the outside world in skin cells or mucous membrane cells or is inside the body in the lining of the lungs, intes-

---

EFA ACTIONS

EFAs are involved in many aspects of normal physiology, including:

- Regulating pressure in the eyes, joints, and blood vessels
- Mediating immune response
- Regulating bodily secretions and their viscosity
- Dilating and constricting blood vessels
- Regulating collateral circulation
- Directing endocrine hormones to their target cells
- Regulating smooth muscles and autonomic reflexes
- Being primary constituents of cell membranes
- Regulating the rate of cell division
- Maintaining the fluidity and rigidity of cellular membranes
- Regulating the flow of substances into and out from cells
- Transporting oxygen from red blood cells to the tissues
- Maintaining proper kidney function and fluid balance
- Keeping saturated fats mobile in the bloodstream
- Preventing blood clots
- Mediating the release of inflammatory eicosanoids that may trigger allergic conditions
- Regulating nerve transmission and communication

For this reason, a diet deficient in either omega-6 or omega-3 EFAs can result in long-term degenerative illness.

tines, or blood vessels—is the body's "first contact" with the outside world and also its first line of defense. The concentrations of the different types of EFAs in the phospholipid layer of cell membranes determines the particular character and function of those membranes. Dietary factors, as we will discuss, can influence these concentrations. Because EFAs are located on the surface of cells, they act as a rapid response team when the body comes under attack, whether from injury or disease. At the localized site of attack, they can be quickly synthesized into eicosanoids (especially prostaglandins) that, among many other functions, initiate the body's inflammatory defense mechanisms. Without this localized response, the body would not be able to call in powerful defenders such as white blood cells to repair an injured area. As we discussed in Chapter 1, the eicosanoids synthesized from EFAs can work to invoke inflammation or to counter inflammation, to cause blood vessel constriction or dilatation, to allow us to feel more pain or less, and much more. They function to balance the intracellular area and ultimately the whole body. Those eicosanoids derived from omega-6 EFAs tend to initiate a pro-inflammatory response, more blood vessel constriction, more pain and mucus, and generally, if overactivated, more disability and disease. Eicosanoids derived from omega-3 EFAs initiate an anti-inflammatory response, reducing swelling and pain and, as we will discuss, promoting health and disease prevention. By seeking to understand EFAs and their influence on cell inflammation and other body functions, we can learn about a biochemical balance that can assist in disease prevention or, when out of balance, can often lead to many of the serious and chronic diseases and conditions that affect modern society.

Omega-6 EFAs

The primary source of omega-6 EFA in the diet is linoleic acid. In the body, linoleic acid is converted to arachidonic acid and other derivatives, which are stored in cell membranes and are used to produce many of the inflammatory eicosanoids (see Figure 3.4 on page 44). The omega-6 pathway, activated by trauma, injury, or chemical stimulus, is the process of converting the omega-6 EFAs found in the cell membranes to these various eicosanoids. If the omega-6 EFA components of the cell membranes become dominant, a pro-inflammatory state can result that may lead to many of the diseases and conditions we will discuss in Chapter 5. For example, arachidonic acid is a particularly common constituent of brain cell (neuron) membranes, and a massive release of arachidonic acid in cerebral cortex ischemia/reperfusion, such as occurs with a stroke, plays a major role in worsening brain damage after the stroke.

Linoleic acid is found in the oils of seeds and grains; sunflower, safflower, and corn oil are particularly rich sources. Evening primrose oil and borage oil are high not only in linoleic acid but also in the omega-6 derivative gamma-linolenic acid (GLA). Avocado also contains a large amount of linoleic acid.

Omega-3 EFAs

The primary source of omega-3 EFA in the diet is alpha-linolenic acid (ALA). In the body, ALA is converted to eicosapentaenoic acid (EPA), docosahexaenoic acid (DHA), and other derivatives, which are stored in cell membranes and are used to produce many of the anti-inflammatory eicosanoids (see Figure 3.4 on page 44). The omega-3 pathway, activated by trauma, injury, or chemical stimulus, is the process of converting the omega-3 EFAs found in the cell membranes to various eicosanoids. If the omega-3 EFA components of the cell membranes become dominant, an anti-inflammatory state can result, with preventive health benefits.

ALA is found in green plants and algae (phytoplankton). The leaves and seeds of the perilla plant (widely eaten in Japan, Korea, and India) are the richest plant sources of ALA. Linseed oil is also a rich source. Fish oil, however, is considered the most important dietary source of omega-3 EFAs because it contains concentrated amounts of the ALA derivatives EPA and DHA. EPA and DHA are found almost exclusively in seafood. The reason fish are so highly concentrated with EPA and DHA is that they are at the top of a food chain based on algae, a single-cell marine organism that manufactures large amounts of EPA and DHA. Small fish eat lots of algae, and the algae's EPA and DHA become concentrated in their fat and organs. Large fish eat lots of small fish, further concentrating EPA and DHA in their own flesh. (This same process of chemicals becoming more concentrated up the ladder of the food chain also can lead to a concentration of toxins such as mercury, lead, dioxins, and PCBs. We will discuss in Chapter 6 how the processing and purification of the fish oil is so important to remove these toxins from fish oil supplements.)

A Change in Our Diet

Modern man may be suffering from diseases and conditions such as heart disease, high blood pressure, stroke, and Alzheimer's disease at unprecedented levels in part due to a major shift in our diet, according to experts such as Artemis P. Simopoulos, M.D., president of the Center for Genetics, Nutrition and Health, located in Washington D.C., and leading authority on how diet affects disease. He and many others point to evidence that our hunter-gatherer ancestors of the Paleolithic period, about 2,500,000 to 200,000 years ago, subsisted on a diet of a variety of natural foods (wild lean meat, fish, green leafy vegetables, fruits, nuts, berries, and honey) that resulted in a balance of approximately equal parts of omega-3 and omega-6 EFAs. During this time, our cells' structure and function

Table 3.3. Omega-6 and Omega-3 Content (as a Percentage) of Common Dietary Oils		
Oil	Omega-6 Content (percent)	Omega-3 Content (percent)
Safflower	75	0
Sunflower	65	0
Corn	54	0
Cottonseed	50	0
Sesame	42	0
Peanut	32	0
Soybean	51	7
Canola	20	9
Walnut	52	10
Flaxseed	14	57
Fish	0	100

Source: USDA National Nutrient Database, online at www.nal.usda.gov/fnic/foodcomp/search

Table 3.4. EPA and DHA content (as a Percentage) of Different Fish Species		
Type of Fish	EPA (percent)	DHA (percent)
Anchovies	5.0	9.0
Cod	1.0	2.0
Cod liver oil	9.0	9.5
Crab	0.2	0.1
Herring (summer)	2.1	2.2
Herring (winter)	1.2	1.3
Mackerel (autumn)	1.0	2.5
Mackerel (spring)	0.3	0.7
Oyster	0.3	0.2
Salmon	0.3	0.9
Sardines	4.0	6.0
Shrimp	0.3	0.2
Trout	0.1	0.5

evolved to make use of a balance of omega-6 and omega-3 fatty acids within our cell membranes.

However, since the beginnings of agriculture approximately 10,000 years ago, with the concomitant introduction of cereal grains as a staple food, this balance has been significantly altered, with a steady increase in omega-6 EFAs at the expense of omega-3 EFAs. This process accelerated about fifty years ago, when cattle began to be fed increasingly on grain (which is rich in omega-6 EFAs) rather than grass (which is rich in omega-3 EFAs). Nutritionists have added to this problem in the recent past by encouraging us to eat margarine rather than butter as a way to avoid saturated fats. But consuming vegetable oil in the form of margarine, made of polyunsaturated fats from grains, has served only to increased omega-6 consumption. Currently, the ratio of omega-6 to omega-3 EFAs in the American diet is 16 to 1 or more. This imbalanced EFA ratio has led to a marked increase in our inflammatory response such that inflammation may persist in a chronic state long after the original stimulus, such as a traumatic injury or disease, is no longer present. Epidemic-like increases in cancer, heart disease, allergies, diabetes, autoimmune diseases, Alzheimer's disease, and other afflictions are in part related to this imbalance. Much of the reason can be found at the cellular level and the way in which omega-6 and omega-3 EFAs exist in a balance in our cell membranes to regulate cellular inflammation.

EFAs in Cell Membranes

Phospholipids and cholesterol are the principal components of nearly all cell membranes. As we discussed in Chapter 1, the fatty acids that make up those phospholipids are predominantly arachidonic acid, EPA, and DHA. When cells are activated by a trauma or other stimulus, these fatty acids are released from the cell membrane phospholipids, and they are converted through the actions of various enzymes, including cyclooxygenase (COX) and lipoxygenase (LOX), to biologically active eicosanoids like prostaglandins (PG), thromboxanes (TX), and leukotrienes (LT).

The composition of fatty acids that make up the phospholipids in cell membranes throughout the body varies considerably. For example, in the brain's gray-matter cells, DHA is the most prominent phospholipid fatty acid. It is composed of hydrocarbon chains that are longer and more unsaturated than those of other phospholipid fatty acids. For this reason DHA can allow for increased membrane fluidity and functionality, which is necessary for the functioning of neuron synapses. However, the composition of fatty acids in cell membrane phospholipids is affected by the supplies of fatty acids that are available. In other words, eating predominantly omega-6 EFAs and only small quantities of omega-3 EFAs will result in cell membranes that contain predominantly omega-6 fatty acids.

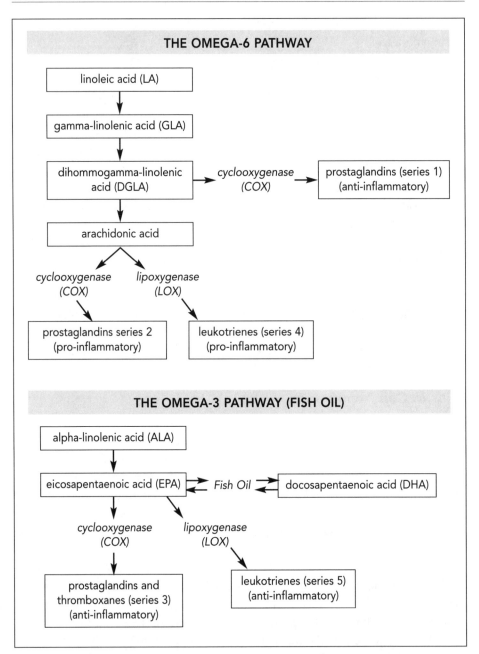

Figure 3.4. Both the omega-6 and the omega-3 pathways require the COX and LOX enzymes to produce prostaglandins (PG), thromboxanes (TX), and leukotrienes (LT). When one type of fatty acid predominates in cell membrane phospholipids, it takes up most of these enzymes, leaving behind little for the other pathway. For this reason, maintaining a balance of omega-6 and omega-3 EFAs is important for optimal biochemical balance in the body.

Table 3.5. Inflammatory Versus Anti-Inflammatory Eicosanoids	
Common Inflammatory Eicosanoids	
PGI_2	Acts as a potent vasodilator
TXA_2	Causes platelet aggregation
	Constricts blood vessels and airways
PGE_2	Enhances vascular permeability
	Initiates fever
	Increases sensitivity to pain
	Recruits inflammatory white blood cells
LTA_4	Causes spasm and contraction of smooth muscle, mainly in the bronchus
	Increases mucus secretion
Common Anti-Inflammatory Eicosanoids	
PGE_3	Decreases vascular permeability
	Decreases sensitivity to pain
	Stops recruitment of inflammatory white blood cells
LTA_5	Causes dilatation of smooth muscle
	Decreases mucus secretion

When cells are activated to release fatty acids from their membranes so that they can be converted to eicosanoids, EPA and DHA compete with arachidonic acid for the COX and LOX enzymes. In this situation arachidonic acid tends to dominate over EPA and DHA for at least two reasons: (1) arachidonic acid is more readily released than EPA and DHA from cell membranes during injury; and (2) arachidonic acid reacts far more rapidly with the COX enzyme than do EPA and DHA. Add these factors to the disproportionate amounts of omega-6 EFAs found in our cell membranes—thanks to the current Western diet—and you can begin to see why chronic inflammation is such a problem in our society.

FUTURE RESEARCH INTO EFAS

The mechanism initially identified as the reason omega-3 EFAs are anti-inflammatory—that they antagonize arachidonic acid metabolism—is probably too simplistic to completely explain their function. It appears that non-eicosanoid-mediated alterations in inflammatory gene expression and an entirely new, recently discovered line of anti-inflammatory mediators are additional mechanisms of action. The current and future research in this area will ultimately show the many diverse and fascinating benefits of using omega-3 EFA supplements such as fish oil.

Arachidonic Acid as a Direct Activator of Inflammation

Arachidonic acid has now been linked to other areas of pro-inflammatory effects besides the formation of eicosanoids. Studies are now underway linking its pro-inflammatory actions directly in fibroblasts, which make up the connective tissues of the body such as ligaments and tendons. Arachidonic acid can also directly activate macrophages and stimulate the production of the markedly inflammatory substance TNF-alpha. Arachidonic acid may be able to regulate inflammatory mediator production on its own, and therefore dietary arachidonic

---

THE ZONE DIET

In 1995 nutritionist Barry Sears wrote the very popular book *The Zone*, which, among several other concepts, discussed the fact that our modern diet had a disproportionate amount of arachidonic acid, and that this had resulted in an overabundance of inflammatory eicosanoids in our bodies. Dr. Sears termed this condition "silent inflammation" and described how this low level of inflammation, from dietary sources, may lead to many of the inflammatory diseases we see today—and that this chronic inflammatory state is rarely noticed until these diseases have taken hold and damage is done. Dr. Sears's proposed diet plan seeks to reduce dietary sources of arachidonic acid and increase the amounts of omega-3 EFAs in the diet, among other dietary changes.

In 2003 Dr. Samuel Cheuvront published an article reviewing the science behind this diet plan. He concluded that a dietary reduction in omega-6 EFAs and an increase in omega-3 EFAs would decrease the amount of series-2 eicosanoids resulting from omega-6 synthesis, thereby reducing the incidence of the chronic health disorders linked to excessive amounts of these eicosanoids.

In 2001 Dr. W. E. M. Lands also concluded that eicosanoids formed from omega-6 EFAs were implicated as mediating inflammation and other conditions since they can enhance clotting, vascular spasm, and heartbeat arrhythmia; worsen asthma; and cause transplant rejection and other immune disorders. His research, and that of many others, including major pharmaceutical companies, has resulted in billions of dollars being spent on new drugs to block omega-6 EFA eicosanoid function. Dr. Lands also foresaw the need for preventive nutrition to cut arachidonic acid in our diets, which would be generally simpler and better than pharmacological treatment for most people.

acid, rather than arachidonic acid stored in cell membranes, can exert a systemic or body-wide inflammatory effect. Dietary EPA, as from fish oil, does not stimulate the production of TNF-alpha or other inflammatory cytokines and may even counter their stimulation by arachidonic acid. In fact, some recent studies now show that EPA and DHA can block the cytokine-induced stimulation of COX-2 production, TNF-alpha, and other cytokines in cultured human osteoarthritic cartilage tissue.

Genetic Responses to Omega-3 EFA

The transcription factor NFκB is located in cell nuclei and is responsible for regulating the expression of genes involved in inflammation, including the production of COX-2, TNF-alpha, interleukin-1, and adhesion molecules. Studies now show that arachidonic acid can directly activate NFκB in white blood cells; this is the mechanism by which arachidonic acid can stimulate the formation of COX-2 and inflammatory cytokines. In contrast, EPA suppresses the activation of NFκB and prevents NFκB activation by other substances as well, so that the formation of these inflammatory cytokines is suppressed. These observations suggest direct effects of omega-3 EFAs on inflammatory gene expression.

New Omega-3 EFA Mediators

Recent studies have identified a new group of mediators, E-series resolvins, which are formed from EPA by COX-2 in the presence of aspirin and can exert anti-inflammatory actions. Studies with DHA have discovered new mediators called D-series resolvins, also produced by COX-2, that also have anti-inflammatory properties. This is an exciting new area of research, and the implications will most likely become very important as a way to explain omega-3 EFA actions.

CHAPTER 4

Fish Oil:
An Omega-3 Powerhouse

On May 27, 2003, John D. Graham, M.D., an administrator within the federal Office of Budget and Management (OMB), wrote a letter to the Secretaries of the Department of Health and Human Services (HHS) and the Department of Agriculture (USDA) urging them to revise the nation's dietary guidelines to include information that omega-3 EFAs have been shown to reduce the risk of coronary heart disease (CHD) and that trans fatty acids, which are found in many processed and fried foods, may increase the risk of CHD.

The text of the letter proceeded as follows:

The purpose of this letter is to request that the Department of Agriculture (USDA) and the Department of Health and Human Services (HHS) further incorporate the large body of recent public health evidence linking food consumption patterns to health and disease as the Dietary Guidelines for Americans is revised for its scheduled 2005 release and to update the Food Guide Pyramid, which was introduced in 1992.

Secretary Thompson [the head of HHS at the time of this letter] has made it clear that both childhood overweight and adult obesity and the associated chronic health problems such as heart disease are widespread in the United States, and have become one of our nation's most important public health problems. However, recent studies suggest that adherence to the Dietary Guidelines has only modest impact on the risk of cardiovascular disease and no significant impact on other chronic diseases such as cancer. OMB believes that these and other studies should play a prominent role as USDA and HHS revise the guidelines. Given the wide reach of the federal nutrition guidelines, we believe that good nutrition habits fostered by improved information on the links between diet and health will have a significant health impact, especially in reducing heart disease. Coronary heart disease (CHD) is our nation's largest cause of premature death for both men and women, killing over 500,000 Americans each year. Even a modest improvement in dietary habits may lead to significant reductions in the number of premature deaths from CHD.

We recognize that the 2000 Dietary Guidelines made some changes in recommendations that may reduce cardiovascular risk. We nonetheless urge you to reconsider all available nutritional and medical evidence as you develop the new guidelines. For example, in a previous letter addressed to HHS, we encouraged the Food and Drug Administration (FDA) to finalize a rule to require a product's Nutrition Facts panel to include the amount of trans fatty acids present in foods. As you know, there is a growing body of scientific evidence, both experimental and epidemiological, that suggests consumption of trans fatty acids increases the risk of CHD. Another important risk factor is the omega-3 fatty acid content of food. Both epidemiologic and clinical studies find that an increase in consumption of omega-3 fatty acids results in reduced deaths due to CHD. The recent revision of the American Heart Association's (AHA's) dietary guidelines recognizes this evidence by recommending consuming fish, which is high in omega-3 fatty acids, at least twice weekly to reduce the risk of CHD. In addition, the AHA recommends the inclusion of oils and other food sources high in omega-3 fatty acids.

The current Dietary Guidelines targets only the reduction of saturated fat and cholesterol, with only a brief reference to the risks from trans fatty acids and benefits of omega-3 fatty acids. We encourage you to consider strengthening the language in the guidance and to modify the Food Guide Pyramid to better differentiate the health benefits and risks from foods. As noted in the Report of the Dietary Guidelines Advisory Committee on the Dietary Guidelines for Americans (2000), consumers find the Food Guide Pyramid to be the most useful part of the Guidelines and the Guidelines itself encourages readers to "let the pyramid guide your food choices." Yet the current Food Guide Pyramid, for example, groups meat, poultry, fish, dry beans, eggs, and nuts into a single "Meat and Beans Group" when research suggests that these foods may not be equivalent in terms of their health effects. Given the significant potential improvement in public health suggested by current evidence, we urge you to consider revising the Dietary Guidelines and Food Guide Pyramid to emphasize the benefits of reducing foods high in trans fatty acids and increasing consumption of foods rich in omega-3 fatty acid.

It could not be said any better! The revised Food Guide Pyramid released in 2005 did indeed describe the need for less saturated and more unsaturated fats. Although omega-3 fatty acids were not recommended on the basis of their merits definitively, the guidelines accompanying the pyramid did cite "limited evidence that suggests eating fish rich in eicosapentaenoic acid (EPA) and docosaheaenoic acid (DHA) may reduce the risk for mortality from cardiovascular disease"—not exactly a glowing recommendation, but a good start!

In Chapter 5 we will see that there is actually much evidence suggesting that EPA and DHA in the diet can reduce the risk of mortality from cardiovascular disease. In addition, these omega-3 essential fatty acids (EFAs), in sufficient quantity, can reduce the incidence and effects of an incredible number of varied health conditions. This chapter will explain why getting a sufficient quantity of omega-3 EFAs through diet alone can be a difficult and potentially dangerous proposition. Plant sources of omega-3 EFAs, such as linseed and algae, simply don't have the quantities of omega-3 EFAs that we require. Fish is considered one of the best sources of omega-3 EFAs. The problem with eating fish as your only source of omega-3 EFAs is that it can contain many toxic substances such as mercury, lead, PCBs, and other contaminants that generally make obtaining sufficient EPA and DHA from fish potentially dangerous. Additionally, most of the studies that have provided evidence for the efficacy of omega-3 EFAs in preventing and mediating disease are based on specific dosages of EFAs that users might like to mimic. For example, the American Heart Association recommends that persons with coronary heart disease get at least 0.9 gram per day of EPA. However, the way fish is prepared and portioned make it difficult for most people to determine how much fish oil they are actually consuming. And cooked fish can contain only a limited amount of EPA and DHA, while the many studies that cite the benefits of these EFAs often used 3 to 5 grams per day in their experimental models.

The solution to these concerns is supplementation with a purified, concentrated, measured source of omega-3 EFAs: fish oil.

WHY FISH?

Is fish oil really the best source of omega-3 EFAs? Absolutely. You could add more omega-3 EFAs to your diet in the form of alpha-linolenic acid (ALA). Good sources of ALA include flaxseed, camelina, chia, perilla, canola, and soybean oils, along with walnuts and arugula. However, the human body converts only about 1 to 9 percent of that ALA to EPA and DHA, the primary omega-3 EFAs for storage in cell membrane phospholipids. It would be difficult to consume enough ALA to raise EPA and DHA levels in the body.

Algae is a good source of EPA and DHA; indeed, it's the dietary source of EPA and DHA for fish. However, it is more difficult and, hence, more expensive to extract these fatty acids from algae and purify them than it is to do so from fish. For vegetarians, nevertheless, it is a viable option.

FISH IN THE DIET

The term *fish* refers to freshwater and saltwater fish, shellfish, shrimp, lobster, and other aquatic animal life. Generally, these fish are highly nutritious foods, full of vitamins, minerals, and high-quality protein, low in saturated fat, and especially good sources of omega-3 EFAs. The problem is that fish can accumulate environmental toxins, such as mercury, lead, PCBs, and dioxins, that can reduce their safety as a food for people.

Nutrition

The amount of omega-3 EFAs that fish contain depends on many factors. Species is an important variable, of course. Herring, mackerel, salmon, sardines, trout, and bluefin and albacore ("white") tuna contain the highest amounts of omega-3 EFAs. The method of preparation is also important. If these fish are cooked under high heat, the amount of EFAs they contain is seriously affected; deep-fried fish, for example, usually has only tiny amounts of omega-3 EFAs, because the frying process transforms the polyunsaturated fatty acids into trans or saturated fatty acids.

Diet is another important factor. The natural diet of wild fish includes algae, plankton, and even other fish, all of which supply EPA and DHA. Farmed fish, on the other hand, are typically fed grain and soy, which are high in omega-6 EFAs, which results in very little of the good omega-3 EFAs in their oil.

Safety

Optimally, we would obtain omega-3s through the regular consumption of fish. However, because of pollutants and contaminants in their water environment, mostly resulting from the fallout of burning carbon-based fuels such as coal and oil, fish pick up many toxins that then become concentrated in their tissues. Mercury and polychlorinated biphenyls (PCBs) are the most common toxins in seafood. Once mercury enters freshwater or seawater, it is transformed into methylmercury by sediment-dwelling bacteria. Methylmercury is concentrated up the food chain as plankton consume those bacteria and are in turn consumed by small fish that are then eaten by larger fish. The toxic effects of mercury can be profound and long lasting, and in some cases permanent. Mercury may cause vague symptoms like fatigue, memory loss, and headaches and can raise the risk of heart disease.

PCBs are colorless and odorless chemicals once used in electrical equipment. Although they were banned in 1976 due to their toxic effects on humans, they can persist in the environment for long periods of time, and most PCBs that entered the environment have ended up in the bottom sediments of rivers, lakes, and ultimately the ocean. Sediment-dwelling organisms ingest these PCBs and pass them up into the food chain in just the same way as they do mercury.

Cooking fish does not remove these toxins. PCBs are stored in the fatty layers of fish, so exposure to PCBs can be minimized by removing the fish skin and

Table 4.1. EPA and DHA Content of Common Seafood

Fish	EPA (mg)	DHA (mg)	EPA + DHA (g)	Total Fat (g)
Bass (striped)	184	637	0.8	2.5
Catfish				
Wild	85	116	0.2	2.4
Farmed	42	109	0.2	6.8
Clams (about 9 small)	117	124	0.2	1.1
Cod				
Pacific	88	147	0.2	0.1
Atlantic	3	131	0.1	0.8
Crab				
Alaska king (about ⅔ leg)	251	100	0.4	1.3
Dungeness (about ¾ crab)	239	96	0.3	1.1
Fish sticks (about 3)	72	108	0.2	10.2
Flounder and sole	207	219	0.4	1.3
Haddock	65	138	0.2	0.8
Herring				
Kippered	825	1,003	1.8	10.5
Pickled	711	464	1.2	15.3
Lobster (northern)	45	26	0.1	0.5
Mackerel				
Pacific and jack	555	1,016	1.6	8.6
Atlantic	428	594	1.0	15.1
King	148	193	0.3	2.2
Mahimahi (dolphinfish)	22	96	0.1	0.8
Oysters				
Pacific, raw (about 1.5)	312	212	0.6	2.0
Eastern, wild, raw (about 6)	228	248	0.5	2.1
Eastern, wild (about 12)	221	247	0.5	1.6
Eastern, farmed (about 9)	195	119	0.4	1.8
Eastern, farmed, raw (about 6)	160	113	0.3	1.3
Perch (Atlantic)	88	230	0.3	1.8
Pollock				
Atlantic	11	383	0.5	1.1
Walleye	157	241	0.4	1.0

Fish	EPA (mg)	DHA (mg)	EPA + DHA (g)	Total Fat (g)
Rockfish	154	223	0.4	1.1
Salmon				
Atlantic, wild	349	1,215	1.6	6.9
Coho, farmed	347	140	1.1	1.0
Sockeye, canned, drained	418	564	1.0	6.2
Coho, wild	341	559	0.9	3.1
Sardines				
Pacific, canned in tomato sauce, drained	520	845	1.4	1.2
Atlantic, canned in oil, drained	402	432	0.8	9.1
Scallops				
Raw (about 6 large)	16	92	0.2	0.7
Breaded and fried (about 6 large)	13	88	0.2	9.3
Shrimp (about 16 large)	145	122	0.3	0.9
Swordfish	111	579	0.1	4.4
Tilefish	146	623	0.8	4.0
Trout				
Rainbow, farmed	284	697	1.0	6.1
Rainbow, wild	398	442	0.8	4.9
Mixed species	220	575	0.8	7.2
Tuna				
Bluefin	309	910	1.3	5.3
White, canned in water, drained	198	535	0.7	2.5
Skipjack	11	201	0.3	1.1
Yellowfin	40	191	0.2	1.0
Light, canned in water, drained	40	190	0.2	0.1
Light, canned in oil, drained	23	86	0.1	1.0
Whiting	241	200	0.4	1.4

Source: U.S. Department of Agriculture's National Nutrient Database for Standard Reference, Release 15 (available at www.nal.usda.gov/fnic/foodcomp/Data/SR15/sr15.html).

any surface fat from fish before consumption. However, this will also remove the fish oil, where the omega-3 EFAs are located. Mercury, on the other hand, is not removed so easily; only a process called molecular distillation, which is performed during the manufacture of fish oil supplements, can extract mercury from fish flesh and oil.

Special Concerns during Pregnancy and Childhood

The conundrum is that the omega-3 EFAs found in oily fish have great health benefits, especially during pregnancy and for young children. As we will discuss in Chapter 5, they are essential for the healthy development of brain, retina, and nervous tissue in the fetus and infant. During pregnancy these fatty acids are transferred from the mother's tissues to the fetus. After birth, the infant's brain and nervous system continue to develop and the infant obtains omega-3s from the mother's milk or infant formula fortified with EFAs. But the toxins found in high levels in fish are harmful, particularly so for a developing fetus or infant. In fact, because of all these toxins, the FDA has strict guidelines for seafood consumption for women who may become pregnant, pregnant and nursing women, and young children:

- Fish that may contain high levels of mercury, particularly shark, swordfish, king mackerel, and tilefish (also called golden bass or golden snapper), should be avoided.

- Total consumption of all other fish should be limited to no more than an average of one serving of 12 ounces (cooked) fish per week; that includes canned tuna fish.

Prior to these recommendations some studies showed that as many as 8 percent of women who became pregnant had elevated blood levels of mercury due to their frequent fish consumption.

The question is how pregnant women and nursing mothers—and indeed all of us—can safely acquire all the health benefits of eating fish without also acquiring all the toxins so prevalent in seafood. These toxins are generally undetectable to the human palate; they do not alter the taste, color, or texture of fish. The answer is simple: fish oil.

FISH OIL: CONCENTRATED, PURIFIED OMEGA-3

As we've seen, omega-3 EFAs are extremely important components of the human diet, and fish is the best source of these EFAs. We focus on EPA and DHA as the primary types of these omega-3 EFAs because they are the most biologically active components of fish oil. The American Heart Association recommends that healthy adults receive 650 to 1,000 milligrams (mg) of EPA/DHA every day, while the World Health Organization recommends consuming 300 to 500 mg of EPA/DHA on a daily basis. Most scientific studies that have seen positive effects from omega-3 supplementation for such conditions as cardiovascular disease, rheumatoid arthritis, osteoarthritis, ADHD, and others used daily dosages between 2 and 5 grams of EPA/DHA.

That's a lot of EPA and DHA! To obtain just 1 gram of EPA/DHA on a daily basis, we'd need to consume quite a bit of fish (see Table 4.2). And as we discussed earlier in this chapter, eating fish in quantity on a regular basis has its own perils, namely poisoning by toxins such as mercury and PCBs. But thanks to modern technology, we have the capacity to extract the EFAs found in fish, so that we can enjoy their benefits while avoiding the toxins. As we learned in Chapter 3, EFAs are the building blocks of fats. When we extract fats from fish, we are left with fish oil, a concentrated solution of unsaturated omega-3 EFAs.

Table 4.2. Amounts of Seafood Necessary to Provide 1 Gram of DHA + EPA			
Fish	**Amount (grams)**	**Fish**	**Amount (grams)**
Catfish	15.0–20.0	Mackerel	2.0–8.5
Clams	12.5	Oysters	2.5–8.0
Cod (Atlantic)	12.5	Salmon	1.4–4.5
Cod (Pacific)	23.0	Sardines	2.0–3.0
Crab	8.5	Scallops	17.5
Flounder/sole	7.0	Shrimp	11.0
Haddock	15.0	Trout	3.0–3.5
Halibut	3.0–7.5	Tuna (canned, light)	12.0
Herring	1.5–2.0	Tuna (canned, white)	4.0
Lobster	7.5–42.5	Tuna (fresh)	2.5–12

Source: Based on USDA National Nutrient Data Laboratory information.

There are now many more than 100 providers of fish oil supplements. Each product is slightly different from the rest, providing different concentrations of omega-3 EFAs. However, the standard 1-gram fish oil capsule contains approximately 180 mg of EPA and 120 mg of DHA. (The remaining volume is usually made up of "marine" oil, which may be a mixture of other EFAs and fatty acids that have come through the filtration and purification process.) Three of these 1-gram capsules would provide 0.9 gram (900 mg) of EPA and DHA, just shy of the daily dosage recommended by the American Heart Association. Supplements with even greater concentrations are available, making it possible to achieve an appropriate daily dosage of EPA and DHA even more easily in one or two capsules.

These supplements concentrate all the benefits of the omega-3 EFAs found in fish, primarily through the "active ingredients" EPA and DHA, without any of the accompanying toxins. This is because the supplements are rigorously purified to remove heavy metals such as mercury and lead, PCBs, and other toxins, as well as to reduce the incidence of rancidity and improve the taste and quality of the fish oil. (For more information on the processes used to purify fish oil, see Chapter 6.)

RESTRICTIONS ON SUPPLEMENT HEALTH CLAIMS

There's no question that fish oil supplements are an excellent source of omega-3 EFAs, and that these EFAs contribute to the prevention and mitigation of a wide range of health conditions. Chapter 5 will discuss the research studies that support this claim, and Chapter 6 will discuss how to use fish oil supplements to address particular health concerns. This information is vital because manufacturers of fish oil supplements are severely limited by government regulations about the health claims—and subsequent specific dosage information—they can make on the packaging of their products.

The Food and Drug Administration (FDA) is the federal agency that regulates dietary supplements and pharmaceutical drugs. It distinguishes between dietary supplements and drugs based on their intended use. The FDA defines a dietary supplement as a product that is intended to supplement the diet; contains one or more dietary ingredients (including vitamins, minerals, herbs or other botanicals, amino acids, and other substances) or their constituents; and is intended to be taken by mouth as a pill, capsule, tablet, or liquid. It defines a drug as a product intended to cure, mitigate, treat, or prevent a disease. Fish oil supplements are strictly dietary supplements, not drugs. As such, the claims that their manufacturers can make for them are strongly limited.

The FDA specifies that while drug manufacturers are permitted to claim that their products will cure, mitigate, treat, or prevent certain diseases, such claims may not legally be made for dietary supplements. Instead, the label of a dietary supplement may contain one of three types of claims: a health claim, a nutrient content claim, or a structure/function claim. Health claims describe a relationship between a food, food component, or dietary supplement ingredient and reducing the risk of a disease or health condition. All health claims must be approved by the FDA before they can be included in product packaging.

In 2004 a fish oil manufacturer submitted to the FDA the following health claim for approval: "A growing body of scientific literature suggests that higher intakes of the omega-3 fatty acids DHA and EPA may afford some degree of protection against coronary heart disease." The FDA interpreted the very positive results of the research supporting this study (all of which is contained in Chapter 5) somewhat more rigidly. Instead of the preceding health claim, the FDA noted on September 8, 2004, that it would allow the following health claim to appear on bottles of fish oil that reported their contents of EPA and DHA: "Supportive but not conclusive research shows that consumption of EPA and DHA omega-3 fatty acids may reduce the risk of coronary heart disease."

It should be noted that the fish oil manufacturer sought only to address a health claim about coronary heart disease. Therefore, other possible health claims about inflammation, pain, dry eyes or skin, asthma, Alzheimer's disease, and so on can all still be submitted to the FDA for review and comment. Until that time, however, other than the above statement, all other claims for fish oil supplements must be structure/function claims, which are limited to describing how a product may affect the organs or systems of the body, without mentioning a specific disease. A structure/function claim does not require FDA approval, but a product label with such a statement or claim must also include a disclaimer that reads "This statement has not been evaluated by the FDA. This product is not intended to diagnose, treat, cure, or prevent any disease."

But as we shall see in the next chapter, treating, curing, and preventing disease are among the greatest benefits of fish oil supplements, with or without government approval of their efficacy.

CHAPTER 5

Fish Oil at Work: Clinical Trials

Over the past 30 years more than 7,000 scientific studies, including 900 human clinical trials, have provided evidence supporting the effectiveness of fish oil and omega-3 EFAs in the prevention and treatment of our most common diseases, including cardiovascular disease, stroke, cancer, hyperlipidemia, Alzheimer's disease, attention-deficit hyperactivity disorder, rheumatoid arthritis, dry eye syndrome, and many other health conditions. The scientific and medical communities, however, continue to resist these facts and pursue strictly pharmacological treatments, instead of also incorporating natural preventive medicine, dietary changes, and behavior modification, which, as you will learn in this chapter, can be just as effective, and in some cases, such as arrhythmia prevention after a heart attack, even more effective. In this section, we will review the investigations that have been made into actions of omega-3 EFAs in regard to various health conditions, and we will learn how important a role omega-3 EFAs play in both the treatment of illnesses and the maintenance of good health.

VASCULAR DISEASE

Since the early 1970s the scientific community has recognized that consumption of omega-3 EFAs from fish oil has significant cardiovascular benefits. Only recently, however, have we discovered the nature of these benefits and how vascular disease in any part of the body, including cardiovascular disease, is associated with inflammation and its negative effects. Here we will look at the very beginnings of this investigation, when Danish scientists H. O. Bang and J. Dyerberg observed a correlation between the low incidence of coronary heart disease among the Inuit Eskimos in Greenland and their high consumption of fish and fish-eating mammals (including seals, walruses, and whales). The Inuit's reduced rates of acute myocardial infarction (heart attack) compared with Western populations was reported around the world and has led to the current explosion of scientific investigation into omega-3 EFAs.

COMPLEMENTARY, PREVENTIVE, AND TRADITIONAL MEDICINES: WHAT ARE THE DIFFERENCES?

The terms *traditional, complementary,* and *preventive* mean many different things to different people. It is important to know the distinctions between them because the way we seek to maintain our optimal health must include knowledge as to what treatments and modalities are available and from whom they can be found.

Most of the world's greatest medical technological advances have been made in the United States, and typically American medical schools teach medical interventions that are considered traditional. Traditional medicine, sometimes called conventional medicine, can be defined as the process of diagnosis and then treatment for a medical condition that has been researched thoroughly. It uses only those treatments that have been proven effective using standards that compare a placebo treatment to the treatment thought to help the condition. This very rigorous standard has led to many lifesaving treatments for many of the world's disease conditions. Traditional medicine places more value on technique and technology than on the inherent healing power of nature, which is considered the central philosophy of many complementary medicine treatments.

Complementary medicine, sometimes called alternative medicine, is made up of a rich array of techniques, modalities, and medical systems that are mostly unfamiliar to the majority of Americans. They reflect the opposite of what medical science provides as "traditional" medicine. This is not to say that these treatments are wrong or harmful, but generally they are not taught, learned, or practiced by traditional doctors. They are, therefore, an "alternative" to what most Americans are accustomed to having as health care. Much of complementary medicine derives from cultures outside the United States or from ancient healing traditions. The more common complementary therapies, such as herbs and dietary supplements, have rivaled traditional medicine's drug industry and result in billions of dollars of sales annually. Worldwide between 65 and 80 percent of the world's population relies on complementary medicine as the primary form of health care. An increasing number of medical schools are now offering courses in complementary medicine for their students; likewise, many hospitals are developing complementary medicine departments.

Many complementary treatments use natural substances such as herbs, botanicals, homeopathics, nutritional supplements, and whole foods. Naturopathic doctors, who are trained to use natural products, believe that synthesized pharmaceuticals are generally more potent and fast acting but also can have unpleasant and sometimes life-threatening side effects.

Preventive medicine is a more recent concept that has its roots in traditional medicine but also often uses complementary medicine. The central concept is to deter the occurrence of an adverse condition or disease. Specialists in preventive medicine are trained in both clinical medicine and public health. They have skills to understand and reduce the risks of disease, disability, and death. Their training is traditional but expanded to also focus on preventive medicine in order to enhance quality of life and continue good health, and not just intervene when disease or disability occurs.

Recently, a new specialty has been developed that takes the ideas of preventive medicine to its natural conclusion: anti-aging medicine. Perhaps vanguards of the next generation of health care, physicians in this field are traditionally trained medical doctors who are additionally certified in the art and science of achieving optimal health and preventing or delaying age-associated disease. An anti-aging specialist has an orientation in preventive medicine, nutritional medicine, and often sports medicine. These doctors are educated in the latest techniques and resources for longevity and maintaining the highest quality of optimum health.

This review is important in understanding where and how dietary supplements like fish oil fit into the bigger picture of overall good health. As a traditional dietary supplement to encourage good health, fish oil is preventive medicine. As a natural alternative to NSAIDs and other pharmacological and medical treatments, it is complementary medicine. And with all the studies now underway to analyze its effects versus a placebo—the type of study considered the gold standard of scientific proof—fish oil is on the verge of crossing over into traditional Western medicine.

Clinical Studies of Cardiac Effects

The number of large, randomized studies demonstrating the positive effects of fish oil is now overwhelming. The importance of these studies, besides the fact that they included large numbers of subjects, is that they were not sponsored by big pharmaceutical companies. In the world of corporate-sponsored pharmaceutical research, drug trials that have positive results are hyped to both the medical community and the general public, but negative results, especially side effects, as we have seen with Vioxx, tend to be buried. We intend to present here the many positive studies showing the effectiveness of fish oils, and also a few that may indicate some caution in a very small, select population.

The story of omega-3 EFAs has been strongly linked to their cardiovascular benefits since the earliest clinical observations were made by the British physiologist Hugh Sinclair in 1944. While visiting a group of Eskimos, Sinclair noted that they lacked any eye changes that would indicate lipid (fat) deposits in their corneas. He found this surprising, since their diet was composed predominantly of the fatty flesh of fish and fish-eating mammals. He also noted that the Eskimos often had nosebleeds. Sinclair knew that fish contained high concentrations of EFAs, thanks to the 1929 work of Evans and Burr. He concluded that Eskimos had diminished fat deposition in their tissues and possibly "thinner" (having an anti-clotting factor) blood as a result of the high concentration of EFAs in their diet. Both of these characteristics, he surmised, would provide significant cardiac benefits. He then further proposed that a deficiency in some EFAs might account for the increasing rate of ischemic heart disease and stroke in Western societies, since the modern diet contained mostly saturated fats.

In the late 1960s Danish investigators H. O. Bang and J. Dyerberg began to investigate the almost total lack of ischemic heart disease in Greenland's Inuit Eskimos. They showed that the distinctive plasma lipid pattern and altered blood clotting of the Inuit was consistent with their low incidence of myocardial infarction (MI), and they attributed these physiological attributes to the Inuit diet. Studies of traditional Japanese populations with high intakes of fish confirmed the findings in Eskimos.

In 1989 the Diet and Reinfarction Trial (DART) randomized 2,033 men from South Wales who had had a recent MI into two different dietary groups: one that ate a significant amount of fatty fish and one that did not. The fish-diet subjects had a 29 percent reduction in their two-year all-cause mortality compared with those who did not eat this diet. Most of the benefits resulted from the reduction of cardiovascular deaths.

In 1999 de Lorgeril and colleagues published the results of a prospective single-blind trial comparing the effect of a Mediterranean diet rich in omega-3 EFAs, consisting mainly of beans and peas, fish, fruit, vegetables, breads, and cereals and low in meat, dairy products, and eggs, to the usual post-infarction prudent diet. Blood tests confirmed that the experimental group consumed significantly less lipids, saturated fat, cholesterol, and linoleic acid but more oleic acids (olive oil) and omega-3 alpha-linolenic acid than the control group. The study was expected to last for five years but was stopped early because the results of the Mediterranean diet were so beneficial. There were twenty deaths in the control group but only eight in the experimental group. Higher concentrations of omega-3 EFAs were confirmed in the blood of all subjects in the experimental group. Follow-up evaluations two years later showed continued benefits of a diet richer in omega-3 EFAs. There were no changes in blood cholesterol or other blood lipids in these subjects.

MAKING KNOWN THE CARDIOVASCULAR BENEFITS
OF OMEGA-3 EFAS

North Americans have among the lowest dietary intakes of omega-3 EFAs in the world. *In fact, it is estimated that 83 percent of Americans are deficient in omega-3 EFAs.* At the same time, it is now known that there is an inverse relationship between intake of omega-3 EFAs and death due to coronary heart disease. Omega-3 EFAs reduce the incidence of coronary heart disease by lowering blood pressure, reducing platelet adherence to the lining of blood vessels, and enhancing blood vessel vasodilatation, among other mechanisms we will discuss. They also protect against and reduce the incidence of coronary events in people with underlying heart disease. A major benefit of consuming omega-3 EFAs is the prevention of ventricular arrhythmia death, including sudden cardiac death, which annually causes some 300,000 deaths in the United States.

The studies we cite here are all large clinical studies that have been published in major medical journals such as the *New England Journal of Medicine,* the *Journal of the American Medical Association,* and *Circulation,* which are peer-reviewed by experts in this field. Despite this publicity, even the most learned and up-to-date medical practitioners are often not aware of the benefits of omega-3 EFAs, and even fewer understand their underlying mechanisms. Knowledge of the benefits of these fatty acids, as based on the strongest and most compelling evidence provided by numerous studies, in reducing the incidence of cardiovascular mortality, myocardial infarction, and sudden cardiac death must be brought from the relative obscurity of a few researchers in the medical community to the general public.

In 1997 Indian researchers undertook a randomized placebo-controlled trial that showed supplementing patients with a recent history of an MI with 1.8 grams of fish oil for one year decreased total cardiac events by 29 percent. Together, cardiac deaths and nonfatal MI were reduced by 48 percent.

Also in 1997, M. L. Daviglus and colleagues concluded a thirty-year study that looked at 2,107 men who in 1957 had been forty to fifty-five years old and were working for the Chicago Western Electric Company. They concluded that the age-adjusted rates of death from myocardial infarction, coronary heart disease, cardiovascular disease, and all other causes were lowest for the men with the highest consumption of fish, with a trend toward lower mortality rates with higher levels of consumption. The men who consumed 35 grams or more of fish per day had a 42 percent lower rate of death from myocardial infarction than those who ate significantly less fish. A similar finding was reported for women in the Nurses' Health Study, established in 1976 by Dr. Frank Speizer, a study which also reported an inverse association between fish intake and cardiac death. Compared with women who rarely ate fish (less than once per month), the risk for death from coronary heart disease was 21 percent less for those who ate fish one to three times per month; 29 percent less for those who ate fish once per week; 31 percent less for those who ate fish two to four times per week; and 34 percent less for those who ate fish more than five times per week. This study involved more than 84,000 nurses aged thirty-four to fifty-nine who were free from cardiovascular disease and cancer at baseline in 1980. The study's architects concluded that among these women a higher consumption of fish (and thereby omega-3 EFAs) was associated with a lower risk of coronary heart disease, and particularly a lower risk of death resulting from coronary heart disease.

In 1999 the Gruppo Italiano per lo Studio della Sopravvivenza nell'Infarto miocardico (GISSI) Prevention Trial randomized more than 11,000 Italian men who had had a myocardial infarction within three months of their enrollment into two groups. In one group, the subjects supplemented with 850 milligrams of fish oil per day, while the control group did not supplement with fish oil. The fish oil group showed a 15 percent reduction in the primary endpoints (death, nonfatal myocardial infarction, and stroke) after 3.5 years, compared with the control group. It is striking that most of the benefit was derived from a 30 percent reduction in cardiac mortality and a 45 percent reduction in sudden death associated with cardiac arrhythmia. Mortality reduction was significant after just three months of fish oil therapy. It should be noted that all other pharmaceutical treatments, including the most common cardiac-disease-preventing drugs such as antiplatelet agents, angiotensin-converting enzyme (ACE) inhibitors, and lipid-lowering therapy, were permitted in both groups.

In 2002 C. M. Albert and colleagues reported on the Physicians' Health Study, in which 22,071 male physicians, who in 1982 were forty to eighty-four years old and had no history of myocardial infarction, stroke, transient ischemic attack, or cancer, were assigned to receive aspirin, beta-carotene, both, or a placebo. Baseline blood levels of omega-3 EFAs at enrollment were found to be inversely associated with the subsequent risk of sudden cardiac death. Men with the lowest levels of omega-3 EFAs had an 81 percent lower risk of sudden death compared to those with the highest levels.

These results are consistent with those of the 1995 study by D. S. Siscovick and colleagues, which also looked at sudden cardiac death in two groups: one supplementing with 5.5 grams per month of omega-3 fatty acids (EPA and docosahexaenoic acid, or DHA), and one that was not supplementing. Supplementation was shown to result in a 50 percent reduction in the risk of primary cardiac arrest. Blood work in this study found that between the two groups, omega-3 levels in red blood-cell membranes ranged from 3.3 percent (the lowest level) to 5 percent (the highest); the higher level was associated with a 70 percent reduction in the risk of primary cardiac arrest.

In 2002 H. C. Bucher and colleagues decided to review all studies that investigated the cardiovascular effects of omega-3 EFAs. They searched the literature for all randomized placebo-controlled trials that compared dietary or supplement intake of omega-3 EFAs with a control diet or placebo in patients with coronary heart disease. Studies had to have at least six months of follow-up data. Added up, these studies had 7,951 subjects in the treatment groups and 7,855 subjects in the control groups. Their findings were consistent whether the omega-3 EFAs came from dietary or nondietary (fish oil supplements) sources. The researchers concluded that a diet supplemented with omega-3 EFAs may decrease mortality due to myocardial reinfarction (MI following an MI), sudden cardiac death, and overall mortality in patients with coronary heart disease.

Coronary–Artery Bypass Graft

An estimated 170,000 Americans undergo surgery for a coronary-artery bypass graft (CABG) each year. This operation, once considered a difficult one, is now almost routine in many medical centers. There is controversy over whether it is now being used unnecessarily to treat coronary disease that could be controlled just as effectively by more conservative, less costly medical therapies. However, many studies have conclusively demonstrated that the operation prolongs life in patients who have a severely blocked left main coronary artery. The surgery is also indicated in most cases in which three major arteries are diseased and for disabling angina that cannot be controlled by conventional therapy. As with any surgical procedure, the operation involves some risk; nationwide, about 1 to 3 percent of bypass patients do not survive the operation or recovery period. One of the most common causes of poor outcomes is blockage of the vein grafts and/or postoperative arrhythmia.

In 1996 J. Eritsland and colleagues evaluated 610 patients who, after CABG surgery, were given either 4 grams of fish oil concentrate per day or no supplement. Their diet and serum phospholipid fatty-acid profiles were monitored to determine whether the fish oil supplement increased the amount of omega-3 EFAs in the membranes of the treatment group's red blood cells. The primary endpoint was 1-year vein graft potency, as assessed by heart catheterization. The study showed not only that the treatment group had fewer vein graft occlusions, but that increases in the omega-3 EFA content of red blood cells corresponded to decreases in vein graft occlusions. The researchers concluded that in patients undergoing CABG, dietary supplementation with omega-3 fatty acids reduces the incidence of vein graft occlusion, and this reduction is dose related.

In a study presented at the 2005 Heart Rhythm Society Scientific Sessions in New Orleans, L. Calo and colleagues reported that taking omega-3 EFAs for a week prior to CABG surgery reduced the risk of developing postoperative atrial fibrillation. Postoperative atrial fibrillation occurs in as many as 20 to 30 percent of patients after CABG, and often this arrhythmia slows the recovery process. The researchers randomized 160 patients scheduled for CABG surgery to either "usual care" or "usual care" plus 2 grams per day of fish oil for one week prior to surgery. They showed that preoperative treatment with omega-3 EFAs reduced the incidence of postoperative atrial fibrillation by more than 54 percent in the patients. In addition, those receiving the fish oil were released from the hospital a mean of 1 day earlier than those not treated (7.3 versus 8.2 days).

In another study presented in 2005 Biscione and colleagues showed that treatment with omega-3 EFAs in pacemaker patients with a history of paroxysmal atrial fibrillation reduced the incidence of subsequent paroxysmal atrial fibrillation by 60 percent. The data suggests that omega-3 EFAs might provide a cost-effective alternative to some types of anti-arrhythmia medications and possibly the placement of pacemakers in certain patients. Additionally, omega-3 EFAs could be used to reduce morbidity and the costs associated with atrial fibrillation.

Restenosis after Percutaneous Transluminal Coronary Angioplasty

One of the most common nonsurgical treatments for opening a partially blocked coronary artery is percutanueous transluminal coronary angioplasty (PTCA). During PTCA, a balloon is expanded into the wall of the blood vessel to reshape it. Long-term benefits of PTCA depend on the maintenance of the newly opened coronary artery. Thirty to 40 percent of patients with successful PTCA will develop restenosis (reoccurrence of stenosis, the narrowing or blockage of an artery) at the site of the balloon inflation, usually within six months of PTCA. Restenosis occurs with a significantly higher frequency in patients with diabetes. The use of stents (small springlike devices) placed with the balloon has reduced the incidence of restenosis by as much as 50 percent, but even with this success, many patients are placed on blood-thinning medication to prevent restenosis following PTCA.

Several randomized placebo-controlled trials have evaluated whether omega-3 EFAs can reduce the incidence of restenosis following PTCA. In the Esapent for Prevention of Restenosis Italian (ESPRIT) Study, published in 2002, A. Maresta and colleagues evaluated 339 patients to determine whether long-term administration of omega-3 EFAs before PTCA would affect restenosis. The experimental group received fish oil supplements containing 3 grams of EPA and 2.1 grams of DHA for one month before undergoing PTCA and for one month afterward, and continued thereafter at half dose for six months. The control group received an olive oil placebo. The study showed a significantly higher rate of restenosis in the placebo group as compared to the fish oil group.

In 1993 J. P. Gapinski and colleagues evaluated four studies that examined the existing evidence for the use of omega-3 EFAs in preventing restenosis after PTCA. They found that in total, there were 14 percent fewer cases of restenosis in subjects who used fish oil after PTCA, as compared to those who did not. They concluded that restenosis after PTCA was reduced by supplementation with fish oil, and the extent of the observed benefit indicated a dose-dependent effect, in that the greater the amount of omega-3 EFAs the subjects were supplemented with, the greater the preventive effect.

High LDL ("Bad" Cholesterol) Levels

Fish oil lowers levels of low-density lipoproteins (LDL) in the blood in a manner similar to the action of statins, a class of drugs that have been used for the past forty years to prevent cardiovascular disease. Statins such as Lipitor, one of the most prescribed drugs in the world, demonstrates a reduction in rates of cardio-vascular death, MI, and coronary stenosis (narrowing or constriction of the arteries of the heart) that cannot be completely explained by their ability to lower LDL levels. As R. S. Rosenson and colleagues reported in 1998, the same holds true for omega-3 EFAs. The beneficial effects of statins and omega-3 EFAs on vascular disease involve nonlipid mechanisms that modify endothelial (blood vessel wall) function, inflammatory responses, plaque stability, and thrombus formation. In 2005 M. Studer and colleagues came to a similar conclusion after looking at more than 275,000 subjects in ninety-seven randomized studies. These studies examined the association between different LDL-lowering inter-ventions and mortality (death) from various causes. The researchers' review confirmed the benefit of statins in reducing the risk of overall mortality and car-diac mortality in patients with or without coronary heart disease. Specifically, they found that statins decreased cardiac mortality risk by 22 percent and over-all mortality by 13 percent, while omega-3 EFAs decreased cardiac mortality risk by 32 percent and overall mortality by 23 percent.

Hypertriglyceridemia

Hypertriglyceridemia (a high triglyceride level) is a known risk factor for cardio-vascular disease. Even with medications and diet modification, hypertriglyceri-demia can be difficult to treat. The medications use to treat hypertriglyceridemia are generally not statins but fibric acid derivatives, such as gemfibrozil (Lopid) and fenofibrate (Tricor), and niacin. However, these conventional pharmaceuti-cal treatments have been found to have serious and unpleasant side effects. Yet more than seventy clinical trials have demonstrated the consistent and potent tri-glyceride-lowering effects of fish oil supplementation. Some studies have shown a triglyceride reduction as high as 79 percent, as compared to a control group.

Combining statins and/or triglyceride-lowering medications with omega-3 EFAs has shown a positive effect in lowering triglycerides in patients resistant to single-drug therapy alone. These studies, however, indicate that a very high fish oil dose may be required to obtain this effect. In one study, adding 3 grams of fish oil to 40 mg of Lipitor on a daily basis reduced triglycerides an additional 33 percent. Another study combined 3.4 grams of fish oil with 10 to 40 mg of simvastatin daily in patients with persistent hypertriglyceridemia, resulting in an additional reduction in triglycerides of 20 to 30 percent.

Other studies have shown that 2 to 4 grams of fish oil alone, in combination with dietary modification, can lower triglyceride levels by 20 to 50 percent in patients with mild or persistent hypertriglyceridemia.

How Omega-3 EFAs Work to Protect against Vascular Disease

Our understanding of the nature of vascular disease has undergone a quantum shift over the past ten years. Prior theory held that vascular plaque, be it in the coronary, brain, or neck arteries, slowly grew over time as fat (in the form of cholesterol and/or triglycerides) was deposited on the epithelial lining and caused a slow, progressive narrowing. When the narrowing reached a critical point, either blood demand would be too great for the vessel to handle and the vessel would rupture, causing a stroke, or, at the point of the narrowing, plate-lets would collect in the narrowed lumen (cavity) and acutely block the vessel, resulting in an acute MI or infarction of brain tissue. The problem is that this theory cannot easily explain why mild to moderate vascular disease with only a limited amount of luminal narrowing sometimes results in an acute MI, nor why progressive lumen-narrowing plaques are rarely the main cause of infarction. These questions and others have resulted in new research that has shown that inflammation plays a key role in coronary artery disease (CAD) and other mani-festations of vascular disease.

As we learned in Chapter 1, a stimulus is required to start the body's inflam-matory reaction, and that reaction is mediated by the immune system and de-signed to identify, react to, and remove the irritant. Therefore a splinter, once it pricks the finger, can cause pain, swelling, redness, and heat. This same process of inflammation is now believed to occur within our blood vessels. We will dis-cuss this immune stimulus, the body's inflammatory reaction, the consequences, and finally how omega-3 EFAs work to block this process.

Vascular disease, the main cause of CAD, is an inflammatory disease in which the immune system is stimulated and so propagates the negative effects of inflammation. The evidence for inflammation's role in vascular disease comes both from direct research and from the indirect evidence that the treatment of elevated cholesterol levels and hypertension that was expected to eliminate CAD by the end of the twentieth century has not occurred. In fact, cardiovascular diseases are expected to be the main cause of death globally within the next fifteen years. The reasons for this dramatic reversal are many, but the root causes are thought to be related to the adoption by developing countries, and by those of eastern Europe, of a Western diet (high in fat and highly processed) and lifestyle (sedentary), which has led to the rising incidence of obesity and diabetes around the world. Cardiovascular diseases cause 38 percent of all deaths in North America; in European adults under the age of sixty-five they are the most common cause of death in men and the second most common cause in women. These facts have led scientists to take a new look at vascular disease, including both its causes and its treatments.

One important factor contributing to the persistence of vascular-related death is the epidemic of obesity. Fat cells, especially the adipose tissues surrounding the organs, of patients with the metabolic syndrome that can cause obesity produce inflammatory cytokines, particularly tumor necrosis factor and interleukin-6. These adipokines (cytokines of the adipose tissue) can affect every cell in the body and can result in increased inflammatory responses throughout the body, but especially in blood vessels.

A report on obese Inuit Eskimos shows that high omega-3 EFA consumption may block these adipokines. Metabolic obesity is very prevalent among the Inuit of Nunavik, who continue to eat a diet rich in fish and, as a result, omega-3 EFAs. As reported by Dewailly in 2001, Nunavik Inuit with predominate abdominal obesity had the typical signs and symptoms of the metabolic syndrome, including glucose intolerance, hyperinsulinemia, hypertriglyceridemia, and low HDL levels. When compared to nonobese Eskimos, those with the metabolic syndrome had significantly greater risk factors for vascular disease, but this same group compared to obese non-Eskimo controls showed significantly higher concentrations of omega-3 EFAs and HDL cholesterol and lower concentrations of insulin and triglycerides. The conclusion was that a higher intake of omega-3 EFAs may attenuate metabolic disorders in obese subjects.

A New Look at Old Plaques

Lipoproteins play a central role in the development of vascular disease. Lipoprotein molecules are made of proteins produced by the liver that link to the cholesterol we consume. There are two main types: low-density lipoproteins (LDL) and very-low-density lipoproteins (vLDL), which carry cholesterol from the liver to the rest of the body. When LDL and vLDL cholesterol levels reach a critical concentration in the blood, the cholesterol is deposited in the walls of blood vessels. High-density lipoproteins (HDL) carry cholesterol from the blood back to the liver, which processes the cholesterol for elimination from the body. Adequate levels of HDL are necessary to prevent excess cholesterol in the blood from being deposited in the arteries. In general, the higher the levels of LDL and vLDL and the lower the levels of HDL, the greater the risk for vascular disease.

Lipoproteins are important in that the lipids they transport are used in many positive ways in our cells, including in our cell membranes and as the building blocks for many hormones. The problem is that LDL and vLDL are small in size, and as they circulate throughout the blood vessels, under certain conditions such as when they are under pressure, in high concentration, or in areas where there are many sharp twists and turns, as is the case in the coronary blood vessels, they can be forced inside the muscle wall (intima) of a blood vessel.

Just as the pricking of a splinter would initiate an inflammatory response in a finger, so the infiltration of vLDL and LDL cholesterol into the arterial intima initiates an inflammatory response in the artery wall. The cholesterol "splinter" results in an enzymatic attack in the blood vessel wall, which leads to the release of phospholipid-produced eicosanoids, specifically the pro-inflammatory series-2 eicosanoids produced from arachidonic acid. Additionlly, the deposition of vLDL and LDL can irritate the smooth blood vessel walls, causing them to become "roughened." This rough surface then produces adhesion molecules by activation of inflammatory genes, thereby attracting more lipids and platelets to infiltrate and adhere to the inflamed blood vessel wall as plaque. The accumulation of lipids then initiates an inflammatory process in the artery that keeps this cycle of plaque formation going. Poorly controlled diabetes can result in similar adhesion, since excessive blood glucose can result in an excessive amount of glucose adhering to and infiltrating the vessel surface, which also activates the inflammatory response.

The intima (the innermost muscular layer of the blood vessel wall) contains smooth muscle fibers that contract to move the blood flow along. The inflammatory response causing the formation of vascular plaque lesions (atheromas) results in asymmetric thickenings of the intima. The arteries are more affected by plaque formation than the veins because the intima is thicker and more pronounced in the arteries, where blood flow is strongest. The vascular plaque lesions can consist of huge numbers of inflammatory cells such as macrophages and T lymphocytes, along with a large lipid pool, very few smooth muscle cells (as they have now been displaced), collagen fibers, and a thin fibrous cap just waiting to rupture to cause an acute blood vessel blockage that can lead to MI or stroke. The inflammatory macrophages and T lymphocytes are attracted to the inside of the blood vessel by the activation of the immune response that was initially stimulated by the lipoproteins that have now penetrated to the intima layer of the blood vessel. They are also attracted by the abnormal surface of the blood vessel in the inflamed area. Once inside, they can stimulate the cytokines, inflammatory prostaglandins, tumor necrosis factor alpha, and other inflammatory by-products. The LDLs, other fats (such as trans fats), and other inflammatory stimuli (such as infection debris) in the vascular system keep the process going. (There is now evidence that poor dental hygiene and dental caries are associated with increased risk of cardiac disease due to the constant flow of inflammatory infectious debris they emit into the circulation system.)

Once started, this cycle of inflammation is continued and strengthened by inflammatory cytokines (such as interleukin-1 and tumor necrosis factor) that call in more inflammatory white cells, alter gene function to increase their own production, and are directly toxic to the cellular membranes. The inflammatory process continues within the plaque until the thin fibrous cap finally ruptures. The contents of the lesion quickly attract platelets, which form a clot, which can lead to the acute occlusion. The weakening of the cap is caused by macrophage cells that have become filled with lipids and form foam cells, which release proteolytic (protein-destroying) enzymes that can break down tissue within the fibrous cap and accelerate collagen degradation. These destructive enzymes, called matrix metalloproteinases and cysteine proteases, are now the focus of major pharmaceutical research because of their ability to destabilize plaques. T lymphocytes also contribute to plaque destabilization by releasing interferon gamma, a protein that inhibits the growth of smooth muscle cells and impairs collagen production.

How Do Omega-3 EFAs Help?

Omega-3 EFAs help protect against vascular disease by preventing and mitigating the effects of the inflammation that results from the infiltration of lipids into blood vessel walls. As we discussed in Chapter 3, when consumed, omega-3 EFAs are rapidly incorporated into platelets and cell membranes and compete with arachidonic acid (an omega-6 EFA) for positions on the membrane phospholipids. Additionally, they compete for the cyclooxygenase and lipoxygenase enzymes, which are catalysts for the transformation of omega-3 EFAs into eicosanoids that are less thrombotic (clot forming) than those produced from omega-6 EFAs. Clinically, this is known as the Inuit effect, as the Inuit Eskimos are known to have a lower platelet count, less platelet aggregation, a longer bleeding time, higher concentrations of prostacyclin (PGI_2, an anti-inflammatory eicosanoid), and lower concentrations of thromboxane A_2 (a pro-inflammatory and pro-thrombotic eicosanoid). Generally, most studies on blood values related to vascular inflammation have not seen significant changes with fish oil supplementation, but EPA/DHA consumption does seem to have an effect on blood lipids, fibrinolysis (the breakdown of fibrin), and the activity of plasminogen activator inhibitor type-1 (PAI-1), a blood factor used to rapidly respond to clots and break them apart.

Since most inflammatory blood markers are not significantly altered by supplementation with omega-3 EFAs, we must look for other theories that may explain the beneficial actions of omega-3 EFAs in coronary heart disease. It is believed that the pro-inflammatory cytokines released during vascular inflammation, or present due to an increased amount of inflammatory lipids, saturated fats, or other pro-inflammatory stimulants, can directly decrease myocardial contractility (the heart's pumping ability) and induce myocardial cell damage by increasing the production of free radicals, thus suppressing myocardial function. Obviously, a reduction in pro-inflammatory cytokine production and increase in anti-inflammatory eicosanoid levels, which is achieved by increasing the amount of omega-3 EFA in the diet, will counter this negative effect.

Another suggested mechanism for the cardioprotective action of EPA and DHA has been attributed to their actions on vascular endothelial cells. Dietary omega-3 EFAs enhance endothelial production of vascular-relaxing factor, which is depleted in atherosclerotic vessels. Improved endothelial function is evident from a recent study that showed that vasodilatation in response to vasodilating drugs is improved in coronary arteries of patients who had received heart transplants and took fish oil supplements for three weeks, whereas vasoconstriction still occurred in the control transplant subjects.

In total, the accumulation of research suggests that the omega-3 EFAs work in several ways to protect against and mitigate the effects of vascular disease, as follows:

- **Inhibit inflammation.** They suppress the synthesis and release of pro-inflammatory cytokines such as tumor necrosis factor alpha, interleukin-1, and interleukin-2.

- **Prevent thrombosis.** They help reduce platelet aggregation (the clumping together of red corpuscles that can form a potentially fatal blood clot in a coronary artery), and promote vasodilation (the dilation of blood vessels).

- **Reduce triglyceride levels.** They lower levels of triglycerides, thereby increasing HDL levels and lowering cardiac risk factors.

- **Prevent arrhythmia.** They help protect against heartbeat abnormalities (like ventricular tachycardia and fibrillation) that appear to be the lethal part of a heart attack.

- **Prevent hardening of the arteries.** They reduce blood vessel endothelium dysfunction by affecting centers within the brain that control the release of hormones (such as cortisol) that can influence the degree of constriction (elevating blood pressure) or dilatation (lowering blood pressure) of the vessel, and enhance vasodilatation locally by the release of the series 3 eicosanoids from EPA and DHA.

- **Reduce inflammatory response in endothelium.** They inhibit monocyte adhesion to the blood vessel walls and thus reduce plaque formation, and suppress inflammatory mediators and thromboxane A_2, an eicosanoid that induces platelet aggregation and vasoconstriction.

- **Reduce blood pressure.** They slightly lower blood pressure, thereby reducing the risk of a heart attack.

- **Reduce blood viscosity.** They "thin" the blood, so that the heart does not have to work so hard to pump blood around the body.

- **Prevent oxidation.** They reduce the formation of free radicals, resulting in less cell oxidative stress, which can lead to cell death and the weakening of blood vessels.

- **Inhibit gene expression of adhesion molecules.** They influence the RNA within cell nuclei to inhibit the production of proteins, such as adhesion molecules, that are associated with blood clot formation.

- **Reduce levels of and stabilize atherosclerotic plaque.** They decrease amounts of plaque (as proven by angiogram studies) in addition to stabilizing plaque structures to make them less vulnerable to rupture; a rupture can cause a clot that leads to heart attack or stroke.

The Tufts Report for the AHRQ

The most comprehensive report and research summary ever done on omega-3 EFAs was prepared in 2004 by Tufts University for the Agency for Healthcare Research and Quality (AHRQ), a division of the U.S. Department of Health and Human Services, and was titled *Effects of Omega-3 Fatty Acids on Cardiovascular Risk Factors and Intermediate Markers of Cardiovascular Disease.* This very thorough 313-page report reviewed the effects of omega-3 EFAs as measured by an incredible array of blood factors, including total cholesterol, lipoprotein cholesterol, cholesteroltriglycerides, apolipoproteins, systolic and diastolic blood pressure, hemoglobin A1c, fasting blood sugar, fasting insulin, C-reactive protein, fibrinogen, factors VII and VIII, von Willebrand factor, and platelet aggregation. They also reviewed the effects of omega-3 EFAs in regard to intermediate markers of cardiovascular disease: coronary artery restenosis after angioplasty, carotid artery intima-media thickness, exercise-tolerance testing, and heart rate variability.

PREVENTIVE SUPPLEMENTATION

The apparent reduction in the numbers of sudden deaths from cardiac causes in observational studies and randomized trials is believed to be due in part to the anti-arrhythmic effects of omega-3 EFAs. Because more than 50 percent of all sudden deaths from cardiac causes occur in people with no history of cardiac disease, preventive efforts with omega-3 EFAs are thought to have a profound effect on sudden death from cardiac causes, at low cost and little risk.

This report was based not on original research but on the results of several hundred clinical studies on omega-3 EFAs. We will review here several of the key areas in the report.

Blood Pressure

The studies that were reviewed found a small but significant reduction in both systolic and diastolic blood pressure with fish oil consumption. The effect was stronger in older and hypertensive populations as well as in diabetics.

Glucose Tolerance

This evaluation was undertaken because of the greater risk of cardiovascular disease in diabetics. Hemoglobin A1c (an indicator of long-term serum glucose levels), fasting blood sugar, and fasting insulin levels were examined to see whether they were affected by supplementation with omega-3 EFAs. The studies that were reviewed showed no significant difference between the control groups and the groups supplementing with omega-3 EFAs. These results are thought to be consistent with the known mechanisms of omega-3 EFAs as potent anti-inflammatory and anticlotting agents; they have not been shown to act directly on insulin or blood sugar levels.

Inflammation and Thrombosis

The major cardioprotective effect of omega-3 EFAs is believed to be their ability to reduce inflammation. As we have discussed, inflammation is the process by which the body responds to injury. Laboratory evidence and findings from many clinical studies have revealed that inflammation is an important cause of atherosclerosis and heart attack. As we discussed above, inflammation can result from small, fatty deposits building up in the lining of arteries. Additional factors, such as being overweight (particularly when the weight is carried around the abdominal organs), leading a sedentary lifestyle, eating a diet rich in saturated and trans fats, diabetes, high blood pressure, infections, cigarette smoking, and chronic and autoimmune diseases, are among the many other causes of vascular inflammation.

The AHRQ report evaluated a common inflammation marker, C-reactive protein (CRP), which becomes more prevalent in the blood during systemic inflammation. Tests of CRP levels in the blood are now used to assess the risk of cardiovascular disease. The high-sensitivity CRP assay was developed especially to predict recurrent cardiovascular disease and stroke, since CRP markedly increases during new coronary occlusion due to angina or acute MI, or reocclusion of coronary blood vessels when an angioplasty balloon or stent has failed. Higher CRP levels are associated with lower survival rates.

The studies reviewed by the AHRQ report found that dietary fish and fish oil supplementation had no effect on CRP levels. This is not surprising, because omega-3 EFAs affect the intravascular surface, reducing vascular reocclusion by blocking the effects of inflammation and not the inflammatory factors themselves. As seen in the 2002 evaluation by Bucher and colleagues of clinical studies (not blood work) of cardiovascular disease, omega-3 EFAs have been found to improve survival rates after an MI.

Intravascular clotting (thrombosis) is the ultimate cause of vascular occlusion (blockage) that, after plaque or atherosclerosis has significantly narrowed the blood vessel opening, results in MI or stroke. It now appears that the cause of an acute MI most commonly is from plaque that becomes unstable and ruptures, which allows the inner contents to be exposed to circulating platelets, which then stick to this area, forming a clot that blocks the blood vessel. As is the case for inflammation, there are blood markers that can measure clotting risk. Of these, fibrinogen, a liver protein necessary for clotting and other blood-clotting factors, has been found to be increased in patients with heart disease and is a predictor of cardiovascular events. And as was the case for the inflammation marker CRP, studies examining blood-clotting markers reported that omega-3 supplementation had no significant effect on these markers. Again, this is to be expected, because omega-3 EFAs are generally thought to work not by reducing levels of clotting factors but by reducing the action of these factors on the blood vessel walls and stabilizing plaques so that they don't rupture.

Cholesterol Levels

The AHRQ report evaluated 182 studies that evaluated the effects of omega-3 EFAs on cholesterol or triglyceride levels in at least twenty subjects. Generally, studies that evaluated overall cholesterol levels showed no significant change with omega-3 EFA treatment. However, omega-3 fatty acids were found to consistently reduce triglyceride levels by 10 to 33 percent. The effect was dose-dependent and found in both healthy subjects and subjects with cardiovascular disease, independent of sex, age, baseline triglyceride level, weight, diet, or lipid treatment. Of particular interest was the fact that many studies showed reduced levels of apolipoprotein B, which is the major protein associated with LDL and vLDL as they circulate in the blood and is known to increase the risk of atherosclerosis.

Clinical Studies

In addition to blood-test studies, the AHRQ report evaluated clinical studies. One of the more interesting reports was from studies that employed the exercise tolerance test. These studies showed that fish oil consumption may benefit exercise capacity among patients with coronary artery disease, although the effect may be small. No theory as to why this was true was related.

One clinical study evaluated heart rate variability, which is an indication of whether a person's heart is more likely to have a ventricular arrhythmia resulting in sudden death. This study showed that fish oil supplementation among patients with a recent MI improves heart rate variability, which may reduce the incidence of ventricular arrhythmias. The same was found to be true for dietary fish consumption in healthy subjects.

Omega-3 Dosing and EPA and DHA Levels

The AHRQ report also evaluated studies that examined whether consumption of omega-3 fatty acids actually changed levels of EPA and DHA in plasma or serum phospholipids, platelet phospholipids, or red blood cell membranes. The correlation between the dose and the change in these factors' EPA and DHA levels appears to be fairly uniform, such that 1 gram supplementation per day of EPA and/or DHA corresponds to approximately a 1 percent increase in the EPA/DHA level in all factors examined. Testing of white blood cell membranes showed a similar increase in omega-3 EFA content after dosing.

AHRQ Report Conclusions

The AHRQ report concluded that there was compelling evidence that fish oils have a strong beneficial effect on triglycerides that is dose dependent and similar in various populations. Fish oils had a beneficial effect on blood pressure, on coronary artery restenosis after angioplasty, on exercise capacity in patients with coronary atherosclerosis, and on heart rate variability, particularly in patients with recent myocardial infarctions. Blood markers for the beneficial effects of omega-3 EFAs were generally unchanged compared to the controls. The amount of omega-3 EFAs in various tissues is fairly uniform. More study, the AHRQ concluded, is needed to assess whether the amount and duration of dosing with omega-3 EFAs is significantly related to their effectiveness on cardiovascular disease.

What the American Heart Association Says about Omega-3 EFAs

The American Heart Association (AHA) has concluded that omega-3 EFAs decrease the risk of arrhythmias (which can lead to sudden cardiac death), decrease triglyceride levels, decrease the growth rate of atherosclerotic plaque, and lower blood pressure. For this reason, they recommend fish oil, through diet or supplementation, for all persons (see Table 5.1).

The AHA also recommends eating tofu and other forms of soy, walnuts, flaxseeds, and canola oil. These contain alpha-linolenic acid (ALA), which can be turned into omega-3 fatty acids in the body.

Table 5.1. Summary of American Heart Association Recommendations for Omega-3 Fatty Acid Intake Relative to the Incidence of Coronary Heart Disease (CHD)	
Patient Population	**Recommendation**
No documented history of CHD	Eat a variety of fish (preferably cold-water, oily fish) at least twice per week. Include in the diet oils and foods rich in alpha-linolenic acid (flaxseed, canola, and soybean oils; flaxseeds; walnuts).
Documented history of CHD	Consume approximately 1 gram of EPA/DHA daily, preferably from oily fish. EPA/DHA capsule supplements may be used in consultation with a physician.
Needs to lower triglyceride level	Consume 2 to 4 grams of EPA/DHA daily in capsules, in consultation with a physician.

STROKE

Around 85 percent of strokes are thrombotic, that is, caused by the formation of a blood clot that blocks the flow of blood through a blood vessel supplying the brain. The antithrombotic properties of the omega-3 EFAs, as described above, can help reduce the risk of this type of stroke. Several epidemiological studies have examined the relationship between fish intake and stroke incidence. In the Zutphen Study, which evaluated fish consumption and the number of strokes in a male population, men who consumed an average of 20 grams per day of fish had about half the number of strokes compared with those who consumed less. Likewise, the National Health and Nutrition Examination Survey (NHANES) epidemiologic follow-up study showed that white females who consumed fish more than once per week had an age-adjusted stroke incidence that was only half that of women who reported not consuming fish. A similar protective effect was seen in both black women and black men. The Nurses' Health Study also reported a trend toward reduced risk for stroke with increasing fish consumption.

In 2005 Belayev and colleagues performed a study with rats that were provided DHA in differing amounts after an ischemic event in which the rats' brain cells were deprived of blood, as they would be during a stroke. As we learned in Chapter 3, DHA is the main EFA component of phospholipid membranes in nerve cells, such as those in the brain. The researchers observed that brain cells lose large amounts of DHA during an ischemic event, and that brain cells depeleted of DHA are almost always the first to die during an ischemic event. But when supplemented with DHA (carried in albumin, a large protein), the rats survived an ischemic event with little or no deficits. The researchers concluded that DHA confers a highly fluid-dynamic state (called plasticity) to cell membranes and is actively involved in the structures of the nerve cell membranes that make up the synaptic and dendritic parts of nerve cells (areas where nerve cells connect to other nerve cells); it can be used to rebuild the phospholipid membranes in nerve cells that are injured during stroke and thus restore injured brain tissue.

C-Reactive Protein and Stroke

As is the case with cardiovascular disease, most of the cellular damage caused by a stroke is due to activation of the inflammatory response. White blood cells are called to the area of brain damage and, in turn, call in the many destructive cytokines we have discussed. Specialized adhesion molecules released by the injured cells allow more white cells to invade the local tissue and accelerate the inflammatory response. The end result is that white cells consume the destroyed cellular debris, leaving the typical hole as seen on CT scans and MRI.

The degree and extent of the inflammatory response to a stroke can be measured by the inflammatory blood marker CRP, which has been shown to be a predictor of survival after stroke. The higher the levels of CRP in the blood, the more massive the injury is, and therefore the greater the likelihood of death. As we reviewed earlier, higher baseline CRP levels can indicate vascular inflammation anywhere in the body, including the brain, and therefore can be a general indicator for higher stroke risk. The Physicians' Health Study measured CRP levels prospectively in 543 healthy men who later developed myocardial infarction, stroke, or venous thrombosis and compared them to a control group of study participants who had no symptoms of vascular disease over eight years of follow-up. Baseline CRP levels were significantly higher among men who subsequently had myocardial infarction or ischemic stroke. Men with the highest levels of CRP had double the risk of stroke as compared to men with the lowest levels. The risk was not modified by other risk factors such as cigarette smoking or abnormal cholesterol or triglyceride levels.

Clinically, supplementation with omega-3 EFAs has been found to reduce the risk of stroke but not to alter CRP levels. As we discussed earlier in this chapter, this finding is not surprising, because omega-3 EFAs protect and limit cell disruption from the destructive effects of inflammation, rather than blocking the inflammatory factors themselves.

DIABETES

Recent studies have shown inflammation to be linked to diabetes. A 2003 report by B. Duncan described a nine-year study of more than 10,000 people who did not have diabetes at the start of the study. The study found that people who eventually developed type 2 diabetes, or non-insulin-dependent diabetes, had increased levels of several markers of inflammation, including C-reactive protein, and that subjects who had or developed higher levels of inflammation markers had two to three times the risk of developing diabetes as subjects with lower levels. A similar conclusion was found by researchers led by P. Dandona from the State University of New York at Buffalo, who found that the latest drugs used to treat diabetes and lower blood sugar levels also resulted in lower levels of inflammation markers.

The association of both diabetes and obesity with an increased inflammatory state can help explain why these conditions are also associated with very high rates of coronary artery disease, heart attack, and stroke. As we know, atherosclerosis (vascular plaque formation) is worsened by inflammatory substances such as tumor necrosis factor alpha, cytokines, and inflammatory prostaglandins. Therefore, inflammatory states associated with obesity and diabetes can result in accelerated and premature plaque formation.

Type 2 diabetes is a leading cause of morbidity and mortality. Prevention of diabetes and its associated burden, primarily cardiovascular morbidity and mortality, has become a major health issue worldwide. Obesity has also become a public health priority, given its growing worldwide epidemic and its vast health consequences.

The research on fish and fish oil supplements for diabetics has focused primarily on the prevention of the potentially severe complications associated with this condition. Early studies on the effects of supplementing diabetics with omega-3 EFAs failed to show any conclusive blood sugar improvement, but many studies have shown a reduction in cardiovascular complications and blood lipid abnormalities in diabetics who eat fish regularly or supplement with omega-3 EFAs. In 2003 F. B. Hu and colleagues at Harvard Medical School evaluated a sixteen-year study of 5,103 female nurses who had had diabetes but not cardiovascular disease or cancer at entry. Over the course of the study there were 362 cases of coronary heart disease (CHD) and 468 deaths from all causes in the study group. The causes of death were CHD or stroke, 161; cancer, 172; and other causes, 135. The researchers noted a strong inverse correlation between CHD and fish intake. Women who consumed fish once a week had a 40 percent lower risk of developing CHD than did women who consumed fish less than once per month. Eating fish five times per week reduced CHD risk by 64 percent and reduced overall mortality by 52 percent. Only fish rich in omega-3 EFAs, such as shrimp, lobster, scallops, and dark-meat fish (mackerel, salmon, sardines, bluefish, and swordfish), showed a beneficial effect. The researchers also calculated the amount of EPA/DHA subjects obtained from their diet and found that study participants with an average intake of just 250 mg per day had a 31 percent reduction in CHD and a 37 percent reduction in death from all causes compared to participants with a low (40 mg or less) daily intake.

In a study published in 1996 involving type 2 diabetics who received either fish oil capsules or olive oil capsules for a six-month period, researchers A. A. Rivellese and colleagues found that the participants who received 2.4 grams of EPA/DHA through fish oil supplementation had a significant decrease in triglyceride concentrations, particularly in levels of very-low-density lipoprotein (vLDL) triglycerides (a reduction of 45 percent). There was also a significant 47 percent decrease in vLDL cholesterol levels and a 14 percent increase in LDL cholesterol. (The small increase in LDL levels is generally not as significant as the decrease in vLDL levels, since vLDL, being a very small molecule, is more likely than LDL to play a major role in penetrating the blood vessel wall and causing localized inflammation that can lead to plaque formation.) There was no

AUTOIMMUNE DISEASES

As we discussed in Chapter 1, the function of the immune system is to distinguish foreign molecules, such as bacteria, from the molecules that belong to the body. The immune system attacks foreign particles by activating the inflammatory response. In doing so, it creates many specialized white blood cells and eventually antibodies that can more easily recognize the foreign invader in the future. In autoimmune diseases the immune system fails to distinguish between self and nonself (foreign), and therefore the body begins to attack itself. Some of the many autoimmune diseases include Crohn's disease, ulcerative colitis, type 1 diabetes, lupus, multiple sclerosis, juvenile arthritis, Graves' disease and Hashimoto's thyroiditis (conditions of the thyroid gland), sarcoidosis, Sjögren's syndrome, temporal arteritis, and various skin conditions. Because the autoimmune conditions are inflammatory and modulated by prostaglandins, omega-3 EFAs have been used with success to reduce the inflammatory response and alleviate symptoms in these cases. Conversely, a diet high in omega-6 EFAs (arachidonic acid) is often associated with worsening of symptoms in these cases.

significant change in blood glucose control and no significant improvement in insulin resistance despite the fact that levels of EPA and DHA in red blood cells increased significantly. Based on these findings, the researchers conclude that long-term fish oil supplementation lowers triglyceride levels in type 2 diabetics without adversely affecting blood glucose control.

RHEUMATOID ARTHRITIS

Rheumatoid arthritis is one of the most common forms of arthritis. It affects 2.1 million Americans (1.5 million women and 600,000 men). Onset is usually in middle age but can occur at any age. Rheumatoid arthritis cannot be cured and has substantial personal, social, and economic costs. The long-term prognosis is poor, with 80 percent of affected patients disabled after twenty years and life expectancy reduced by an average of three to eighteen years. The medical cost of rheumatoid arthritis averages $5,919 per case per year in the United States as reported in 1999. Current antirheumatic drugs have limited efficacy and many side effects and, due to the progressive nature of the disease, do not improve the long-term prognosis of patients.

Rheumatoid arthritis is characterized by inflammation of the synovium (the membrane lining of a joint), which causes pain, stiffness, warmth, redness, and swelling. The synovial membrane undergoes chronic inflammatory changes including reactive tissue growth, an increase in the number of blood vessels in the joint tissue, and infiltration by inflammatory white blood cells. Excess levels of inflammatory substances such as tumor necrosis factor alpha, interleukin-6, interleukin 1(b), and leukotriene B4 are present in the synovial fluid. As the disease progresses the inflammation can spread to the surrounding bone and cartilage, causing the characteristic deformities often seen in the finger joints. Although the inflammatory response has been classified in the past as autoimmune, the latest studies indicate there may be antigens in the synovial fluid, which has led to the theory that an exogenous (outside of the body) antigen, such as a viral protein, may be stimulating the immune inflammatory response.

Dozens of clinical studies have revealed the benefits of fish oil supplementation in alleviating the inflammation symptoms of rheumatoid arthritis, showing that fish oil reduces levels of inflammatory cytokines in the synovial fluid by up to 90 percent. In 1995 J. M. Kremer and colleagues conducted a double-blind, placebo-controlled study that showed that fish oil supplementation of 130 mg per kilogram per day decreased the number of tender joints, the duration of morning stiffness, and overall pain in patients with rheumatoid arthritis.

Fish oil supplementation is often trialed to evaluate its ability to relieve pain and, as a result, reduce the use of nonsteroidal anti-inflammatory drugs (NSAIDs). For example, in 1993 C. S. Lau and colleagues compared the supplementation of 2.8 grams of fish oil daily versus a placebo in 64 patients with stable rheumatoid arthritis. In three months the fish oil group showed significant reduction of NSAID use as compared with the placebo group, and that reduction peaked at twelve months.

The ability of omega-3 EFAs to reduce the inflammatory response is the main mechanism of symptom reduction for many types of arthritis. A concurrent reduction in the amount of dietary omega-6 EFAs has been shown to have an additive effect, yielding additional improvements. In 2000 D. Volker and colleagues demonstrated that lower doses of fish oil (about 2.3 grams) could have the same effect as higher levels if the diet was altered to contain only low amounts of omega-6 EFAs. The positive effects were most pronounced three months after the trial began.

In patients with severe symptoms of arthritis, which often result in deformity, other more powerful drugs such as corticosteroids are often prescribed. As we have learned, these powerful drugs can have serious side effects and can lead to bone loss, suppressed immune function, and increased blood sugar levels. In 2003 O. Adam showed that the use of both NSAIDs and steroids could be reduced through supplementation with omega-3 EFAs, and that the use of these drugs could be reduced even further if the patient consumed lesser amounts of omega-6 EFAs.

Although omega-3 EFAs are not a cure for rheumatoid arthritis, these and other studies show us that fish oil supplementation has the potential to reduce or even eliminate the need for NSAIDs. And considering the many serious side effects seen with prolonged NSAID use, as we reviewed in Chapter 2, such supplementation may offer persons with rheumatoid arthritis a significantly better way to manage their symptoms. Proper dosing is based on symptom improvement. Since symptom improvement may not be noticeable until up to three months after starting omega-3 EFA supplementation, determining the proper dose can be difficult. Several studies on rheumatoid arthritis have shown an effective dose range of 2 to 6 grams of fish oil per day.

Rheumatoid arthritis is also associated with an increased risk of cardiovascular disease and osteoporosis due in part to the action of matrix metalloproteinases (MMP), which are found in increased levels in the joint synovial fluid and in the systemic circulation of patients with rheumatoid arthritis. MMPs are proteolytic, which means they can break apart protein bonds. Because MMPs can destabilize vascular plaque in the blood, they may lead to an increased risk for myocardial infarction in people with rheumatoid arthritis. In the joint space, they invade the synovial tissue in cartilage and cause cartilage destruction and bone erosion. Bone tissue is also destroyed via the action of white blood cells activated by the chronic inflammation; they either consume bone directly or stimulate osteoclasts (specialized cells that remodel bone) to absorb the bone. The use of omega-3 EFAs by patients with rheumatoid arthritis is believed to reduce joint destruction caused by MMPs and also to counteract the adverse cardiac effects of the blood-borne MMPs, thereby reducing the incidence of heart attack.

SPINE PAIN

Degenerative disc disease is one of the greatest causes of pain and disability in the United States. It affects approximately one out of four people at some time in their lives. This "wear and tear" condition is most often treated initially with NSAIDs. But as we have learned, this may not be the ideal treatment for a progressive and chronic problem that can last months or years. Because of our research on fish oil supplements with omega-3 EFAs, we concluded that people could use them as a safe and effective alternative to NSAIDs for the treatment of pain. Based on this belief, we undertook an evaluation of people who complained of neck and low-back pain from disc and arthritic causes who had been seen in our practice and had recently been started on fish oil supplements.

In this study, we surveyed 125 people who had been taking NSAIDs who were asked to take a fish oil supplement with at least 1 gram of omega-3 EFAs in the form of EPA and DHA for their symptoms of neck and low-back pain. The results showed that 60 percent of those surveyed experienced an improvement in overall pain, and 59 percent discontinued use of NSAIDs and were using only fish oil to control their pain. This study also found that most patients had no significant side effects and 88 percent planned to continue the use of omega-3 EFAs.

This study was presented to a national meeting of neurosurgeons and was presented a first-place award. It has now been published in the peer-review journal *Surgical Neurology*. This information will now be available to neurosurgeons around the world who had only known of the pharmaceutical treatments for this condition.

OSTEOARTHRITIS

Osteoarthritis, sometimes described as "wear and tear arthritis," is more common than rheumatoid and is also an inflammatory condition of the joints that can be painful, deforming, and disabling. It is caused by the gradual destruction over time of joint cartilage, which is the cushion between bones that prevents them from grinding against each other. It can affect any joint in the body and is the most common reason for major joint replacement, such as of the hip or knee. It also commonly affects the spine, resulting in severe disability and pain.

Because osteoarthritis was thought to be progressive and an inevitable result of aging, research into the possible benefits of treating this disease with omega-3 EFAs was limited. Only recently did evidence begin to emerge suggesting that omega-3 EFAs could alleviate some symptoms of osteoarthritis. In 1998 research undertaken by a team at Cardiff University demonstrated that omega-3 EFAs not only could relieve the inflammation associated with this disease but also could switch off the aggrecanases and other collagen-degrading enzymes that break down joint cartilage. And in 2004 C. L. Curtis and colleagues demonstrated that when omega-3 EFAs were placed with inflammatory cytokines in cartilage cultures, they protected the cartilage from breakdown.

INFLAMMATORY BOWEL DISEASE

Inflammatory bowel disease is the name for either of two autoimmune disorders that cause the intestines to become inflamed: Crohn's disease and ulcerative colitis. These conditions are generally chronic, but they have periods of remission as well as periods of acute inflammation, with associated abdominal pain and abnormal stools. More than 600,000 Americans have inflammatory bowel disease diagnosed every year. Ulcerative colitis is a chronic inflammation of the large intestine (colon). In patients with ulcerative colitis, ulcers and inflammation of the inner lining of the colon lead to symptoms of abdominal pain, diarrhea, and rectal bleeding. Crohn's disease is generally more intense than ulcerative colitis and causes ulcers all along the length of the small and large intestines as a result of severe inflammation.

The standard treatments for inflammatory bowel disease mostly involve powerful steroids, which can have serious side effects. For this reason, sufferers of these conditions have embraced the natural alternatives of supplementing with omega-3 EFAs to take advantage of their potent anti-inflammatory properties and modifying their diet to reduce the amount of omega-6 EFAs they consume. Studies examining omega-3 supplementation and dietary modification have shown them both to be effective in alleviating the symptoms of these conditions. The tendency of all studies was to treat with higher amounts of EPA and DHA (3 to 6 or more grams per day) in order to achieve symptom improvement. However, while the effects of omega-3 EFA supplementation have been found to alleviate the symptoms of inflammatory bowel disease, this therapy is most beneficial because it allows sufferers to reduce the dosages of drugs (steroids) generally required to control symptoms.

E. Ross in 1993 and Y. I. Kim in 1996 both found fish oil therapy to have significant beneficial effects on symptoms associated with inflammatory bowel disease. They concluded that fish oils may exert their beneficial effects by shifting eicosanoid synthesis to less inflammatory species and by modulating tissue levels of inflammatory cytokines.

A 1997 study by M. A. French and colleagues showed that increasing dietary omega-3 EFA intake in patients with inflammatory bowel disease enhanced by 65 percent their absorption and the utilization of saturated fatty acids such as palmitic acid, which improved their overall nutritional status. Several randomized, double-blind, placebo-controlled crossover trials of fish oil have indicated a beneficial effect in ulcerative colitis. In 1992 W. F. Stenson reported that supplementation with 5.4 grams of EPA and DHA from fish oil resulted in reduced levels of omega-6-derived pro-inflammatory eicosanoids in subjects with ulcerative colitis. Also in 1992, A. B. Hawkins and colleagues reported that treatment of inflammatory bowel disease with 4.5 grams of EPA and 1.1 grams of DHA resulted in a significant reduction in steroid intake and a trend toward remission, but it had no effect in the rate of relapse.

In 1990 P. Salomon and colleagues studied the effects of supplementing Crohn's sufferers with 4.5 grams of EPA and DHA from fish oil daily; after two months, the subjects reported a 70 percent improvement in their symptoms and an 80 percent reduction in their use of steroid medication. These results, along with the 1996 report from R. Shoda and colleagues that showed an increased incidence of Crohn's disease in Japan is correlated with an increased intake of omega-6 EFAs, suggest a role for omega-3 EFAs in the prevention and treatment of Crohn's disease.

SYSTEMIC LUPUS ERYTHEMATOSUS

Systemic lupus erythematosus (SLE) is an autoimmune disease that affects a half to 2 million people in the United States, of which 80 to 92 percent are women. SLE affects primarily the joints, skin, kidneys, lungs, heart, and intestinal tract. This condition is characterized by a rash on the nose and cheeks, sun sensitivity, arthritic symptoms, and blood abnormalities such as anemia and positive markers for autoimmune diseases such as LE prep, anti-DNA, and positive ANA test (blood tests that can measure the amount of immune activity in the body and whether the immune system is responding inappropriately by attacking itself).

The common pharmaceutical treatments are powerful immunosuppressive drugs such as steroids, NSAIDs, and occasionally chemotherapy drugs, all of which can have significant side effects. Early animal studies using fish oil on autoimmune-diseased mice consistently showed beneficial effects such as delayed onset of lupus-induced kidney disease; decreased levels of anti-DNA antibodies, which are commonly measured to assess the severity of lupus; and decreased levels of pro-inflammatory cytokines, which are generally markedly increased with lupus. In 2000 B. O. Lim and colleagues compared supplementation with omega-6 EFAs (corn oil) to supplementation with omega-3 EFAs in rats with a suppressed immune system (a clinical effect similar to that of lupus in humans) and found that the omega-3 supplementation caused elevated levels of antioxidant enzymes, decreased levels of pro-inflammatory cytokines, reduced incidence of renal disease, and prolonged life span as compared to the corn oil group. In 2004, in one of the best placebo-controlled studies, Duffy and colleagues evaluated fifty-two patients with systemic lupus erythematosus divided into two groups: one taking 3 grams of EPA daily and one taking a placebo. The study lasted twenty-four weeks and participants were assessed at the start and at six, twelve, and twenty-four weeks. The researchers found that disease activity at twenty-four weeks, as measured by the systemic lupus activity measure (SLAM-R) score, was significantly less in the group that had supplemented with fish oil than in the placebo group. The fish oil group had a significant decline in systemic lupus activity. The researchers concluded that supplementation with fish oil may be effective in favorably modifying the symptomatic disease activity in lupus.

MULTIPLE SCLEROSIS

Multiple sclerosis (MS) is an inflammatory, autoimmune, demyelinating disease of the central nervous system. It commonly occurs at an early age, most often in the early adult years. Its most frequent symptoms include numbness of the legs and arms, impaired vision, loss of balance, weakness, bladder dysfunction, fatigue, and psychological changes. The disease can wax and wane for many years, but in about half of all cases it steadily progresses to severe disability and premature death. This disease is characterized by T cells and other immune and inflammatory mediators entering the brain and attacking the nerve cells, stripping away the nerve cells' myelin sheath and destroying their axons, leaving plaquelike scars. An MRI of the brain is the best test to diagnosis MS, as it can pick up the characteristic "white-matter plaques" that are seen in the white matter or nerve-sheath areas of the brain.

The cause of MS is not known, but various theories about its identity exist, including infection, genetics, and pollution and environmental toxins. Drug therapies for MS are highly toxic, including immunosuppressant steroids and the chemotherapy drugs methotrexate and cytoxan. In 1993 interferon ß-1b was approved in the United States as a suppression therapy to blunt the autoimmune response, but this drug itself is a very expensive drug that requires an injection and is associated with frequent and severe adverse effects. The limitations of the conventional drug therapies for MS have led many researchers to look for alternatives, including supplementation with fish oil.

Diet has recently been the subject of study to determine whether it plays a role in the disease's initiation or progression. Diets high in animal (saturated) fats and certain food allergies have both been found to "trigger" MS flare-ups.

As early as 1952, R. L. Swank and colleagues found that, in Norway, inland farming communities had a higher incidence of MS than coastal communities. Further studies showed that, comparatively, the inland diet contained much more animal and dairy products and the coastal diet contained much more cold-water fish. The researchers reported a strong positive association between butterfat consumption and MS incidence, and a strong negative association between fish consumption and MS. In 1974 B. W. Agranoff and D. Goldberg found an extremely high correlation between milk consumption and MS, and a lower incidence of MS with increasing fish and vegetable consumption in the American population. The same has now been shown to be true for populations of twenty other countries. Food allergies, especially to gluten, sulfite additives, and milk products, have also been linked to the development of MS and the worsening of MS symptoms.

The pro-inflammatory Western diet, with its high content of animal fats and omega-6 EFAs and low content of the anti-inflammatory omega-3 EFAs DHA and EPA, is believed by some to be one of the major factors influencing MS. As discussed earlier in regard to stroke, the delicate endothelial lining of the blood vessels is vulnerable to pro-inflammatory attack, and inflammation of blood vessels in the brain is characteristic of MS. Hardened areas, called plaques (not to be confused with plaques that can occur in the lining of blood vessels), frequently arise around venous blood vessels in the brain that are actively inflamed and have the associated platelet accumulation. As with cardiovascular disease and stroke, omega-3 EFAs will help balance this inflammation, allowing the body to heal the supporting myelin sheaths and nerve cell membranes.

ASTHMA

Asthma is a chronic inflammatory disease that causes the airways of the lungs to be hyper-responsive to cold, smoke, allergens, infections, and other irritants. It is characterized by symptoms such as wheezing and coughing and is also typically associated with airflow obstruction that is often reversible either spontaneously or with treatment. Because of asthma's inflammatory nature, the drugs used to treat the condition are generally powerful anti-inflammatories such as steroids, which are associated with serious side effects.

Asthma is a major public health problem in developed countries, especially in children. Over the past few decades its incidence has increased dramatically. The reasons for this increase are not known, but a number of environmental factors, including air pollution, cigarette smoking, allergies, and diet, have been proposed as potential causes. However, some researchers have found that dietary changes, especially the reduction of fresh fruit and vegetables and the rise of saturated fats over polyunsaturated fats, may be the cause for the rise in incidence of asthma. In fact, recent research has shown that pro-inflammatory leukotrienes derived from the arachidonic acid (omega-6) pathway are one of the major causes of airway inflammation, and the newest class of leukotriene modifiers has been proven very effective in relieving symptoms in asthmatics.

Since increased omega-3 EFA intakes are known to decrease the amount of arachidonic acid available for the formation of inflammatory mediators, a number of clinical trials have examined the effects of omega-3 EFA supplementation in asthmatic individuals. Although there is some evidence that omega-3 EFA supplementation can decrease the production of inflammatory mediators in asthmatic patients, evidence that it decreases the clinical severity of asthma in controlled trials has been inconsistent. The conclusion has generally been that omega-3 EFA supplementation is best used as an adjunct to conventional pharmacologic treatments for asthma.

There is, however, stronger evidence to suggest that omega-3 EFAs are potent at blunting the allergic sensitization that is sometimes the underlying stimulus for asthma. The mechanism for this is that omega-6 EFA consumption increases levels of the inflammatory prostaglandin E_2, which in turn promotes thromboxane A_2, which can stimulate the formation of immunoglobulin E (IgE). IgE is an antigen-specific protein, meaning that it reacts to very specific stimuli, such as pollen, hay, pet dander, and so on, that are commonly associated with inducing an asthma attack. IgE interacts with mast cells and eosinophils, which release the substances responsible for airway constriction and increase mucus secretion. IgE is also responsible for typical skin allergy or immediate hypersensitivity reactions, such as hives and anaphylaxis. By increasing the amount of omega-3 EFAs and thereby decreasing the amount of omega-6 EFAs available to produce IgE, fish oil can help reduce airway reactivity and hypersensitivity. This effect is also the main reason why allergic skin conditions are improved with omega-3 EFA supplementation.

The use of omega-3 EFA supplementation in asthma was sparked by Horrobin's study in 1987, which noted the low incidence of asthma in Eskimos and concluded that it stemmed from their consumption of large quantities of oily fish. Additional research has indicated that omega-3 EFAs have some protective and even therapeutic effect through their impact on mediators of inflammation. In 1998 Hodge and colleagues reported on the incidence of asthma in 574 children. They found that those children who ate oily fish high in omega-3 EFAs, such as sardines, tuna, and salmon, were significantly less likely to have asthma compared to those who did not. They found that the diet of the children who had asthma did not differ from that of the nonasthmatic children in any other regard, and a protective effect was not seen with other types of fish. The benefit of the fish was thought to be due to the ability of omega-3 EFAs to mitigate allergic sensitization, rather than their direct effect on asthma; however, more recent studies report that omega-3 EFAs can reduce bronchial inflammation and therefore reduce the frequency of asthmatic attacks.

In 2004 R. K. Woods and colleagues looked at 1,600 asthmatic adults with an average age of thirty-four years and found, through blood tests and questionnaires, that those who had higher levels of the pro-inflammatory omega-6 EFAs were more likely to have an increased severity of their asthma compared to those with lower levels. This study supports the belief that the types of dietary fats being consumed can affect asthma severity.

DRY EYE SYNDROME

Dry eye is one of the most common conditions of the eyes. It affects approximately 14 percent of people over the age of forty, and its prevalence increases with age. There are many causes of dry eyes, including long-term contact lens wear, LASIK eye surgery, certain viral infections of the cornea, and diabetes. Anything that decreases tear production or increases tear evaporation may cause dry eye. Diabetes, for example, can cause a loss of corneal sensation; this numbness on the surface of the eye can cause the eye not to react to normal stimuli that encourage the formation of tears, resulting in dry eye irritation and inflammation of the eye tissues.

Tears are a salt solution that supply the eye with oxygen and electrolytes. (The eye has no direct blood supply.) The tear layer is covered by a layer of oil, produced by the oil glands in the eyelid, that protects it from evaporation. When the eye becomes dry, the tears lose water and become too salty, which results in a stinging and burning sensation on the eye surface. A temporary treatment is saline eye drops, or artificial tears, which are designed to cover up the dry spots on the eye. However, if the content of the artificial tears does not precisely match the body's electrolyte (sodium and potassium) balance, the drops can deplete the levels of electrolytes on the surface of the eye and actually decrease the quantity of lubrication, exacerbating the problem.

Research presented for the first time at the 2003 annual meeting of the Association for Research in Vision and Ophthalmology showed that a high dietary intake of omega-3 EFAs decreases the risk of dry eye. Using the Women's Health Database at the Harvard School of Public Health, the investigators examined the dietary intake of EFAs in 32,470 female health professionals. They found that the higher the ratio of dietary omega-3 to omega-6 EFAs, the lower the likelihood of dry eye; and the lower the ratio of omega-3s to omega-6s, the higher the likelihood of dry eye. They found that, in general, the higher the intake of omega-3 EFAs, the lower the likelihood of dry eye.

The omega-3 EFAs help provide relief for dry eye syndrome by suppressing inflammation and providing the oil glands in the eyelid with the building blocks they need to manufacture the oil film over the tear layer. As we have noted, omega-3 EFAs in the diet are incorporated into cell membranes and, from there, can be transformed by enzymes into anti-inflammatory eicosanoids such as prostaglandin E_3 (PGE₃) and leukotriene B_5 (LTB₅). Even more important for dry eye and other inflammatory eye conditions is the fact that omega-3 EFAs can block the gene expression of the powerful inflammatory cytokines tumor necrosis factor alpha (TNF-α), interleukin-1 alpha (IL-1α), and leukin-1 beta (IL-1β). Suppressing TNF-α is important especially in Sjögren's syndrome, a chronic disorder that causes insufficient moisture production in certain glands of the body. Sjögren's syndrome is an autoimmune disease in which the immune system attacks and destroys moisture-producing glands, including salivary glands and lacrimal (tear-producing) glands, which can cause severe dry eyes with burning and chronic redness. In this inflammatory condition, increased TNF-α in the lacrimal glands increases lacrimal gland apoptosis (programmed cell death). Increased apoptosis contributes to the decrease in tear production. In addition, TNF-α induces apopotosis on the surface of the dry eye, which can lead to the chronic redness and irritation.

MACULAR DEGENERATION

Macular degeneration is a degenerative eye disease that affects more than 10 million Americans. It is the leading cause of legal blindness in persons over the age of fifty-five in the United States. While painless, macular degeneration often interferes with reading, driving, and other daily activities. There are two forms of macular degeneration. Dry macular degeneration affects about 90 percent of those with the disease and causes gradual loss of central vision, initially only in one eye. Wet macular degeneration, which accounts for 90 percent of all severe vision loss from the disease, involves a very sudden loss of central vision. Dry macular degeneration occurs from the breakdown of the light-sensitive cells in the center of the retina, called the macula. Wet macular degeneration occurs when new blood vessels behind the retina grow toward the macula and leak blood and fluid. Along with antioxidants, such as carotenoids, zeaxanthin, lutein, selenium, zinc, and vitamins C and E, that have been shown to protect the retina, omega-3 EFAs have been studied and used to delay or prevent macular degeneration.

In 2003 J. P. SanGiovanni and colleagues reported on the Age-Related Eye Disease Study, a study undertaken by the National Eye Institute involving 4,513 sixty- to eighty-year-olds. Those subjects who ate fish more than twice a week were half as likely to get macular degeneration as those who ate no fish at all. More than one weekly portion of broiled/baked fish or canned tuna lowered the risk by a third. Also in 2003, J. M. Seddon evaluated 261 patients with acute macular degeneration and found that higher levels of certain dietary fats were associated with the progression of the degeneration to the advanced stages, which often involve visual loss. The study found that a higher intake of vegetable fat and, to a lesser extent, animal fat increased the rate of progression. The researchers concluded that fish and nut consumption reduced the risk of progression.

ECZEMA

Eczema describes a skin condition that causes an itchy, inflamed rash. Atopic dermatitis, a form of eczema, is a noncontagious disorder, often associated with stress and allergies, that is characterized by chronic inflammation of the skin and can cause intolerable itching. Atopic dermatitis is most common in infants, children, and young adults. While allergic reactions often trigger atopic dermatitis, the condition can also result from an overactive immune response in which the immune system, including white blood cells, cytokines, and inflammatory eicosanoids, causes the skin to lose abnormally large amounts of moisture. The condition can be aggravated by a cycle that develops in which the skin itches, the patient scratches, the condition worsens, the itching worsens, the patient scratches, et cetera. This cycle must be broken by relieving the itching to allow the skin time to heal. If the skin becomes broken, the risk of developing a skin infection exists.

As you might expect, due to their anti-inflammatory effects, omega-3 EFAs have been shown to significantly alleviate atopic dermatitis in a number of clinical trials. In 1994 E. Soyland and colleagues evaluated 145 patients with atopic dermatitis who were randomly assigned to receive 6 grams per day of either fish oil (omega-3 EFAs) or corn oil (omega-6 EFAs). The results showed improvement in 30 percent of the fish oil group compared to 24 percent of the corn oil group. In the fish oil group, the amount of omega-3 EFAs in the membranes of red blood cells was significantly increased at the end of the trial, whereas the level of omega-6 EFAs was decreased.

PSORIASIS

Psoriasis is a chronic inflammatory skin disease that is characterized by distinct, red, scaly patches on the body and scalp. The lesions may itch, sting, and occasionally bleed. Psoriasis can also lead to a severe form of arthritis. This disease affects 1 to 2 percent of the general population. About a third of people with psoriasis have a family history of psoriasis, but physical trauma, acute infection, and some medications are believed to trigger the condition. A 1988 study by S. B. Bittiner and colleagues found that daily supplementation with 10 grams of fish oil lessened the severity of skin lesions. In 1989 C. E. Dewsbury and colleagues found that applying a topical preparation containing 10 percent fish oil directly to psoriatic lesions twice daily resulted in improvement after seven weeks. A 1991 trial by T. Kojima and colleagues found that 3.6 grams per day of EPA reduced the severity of psoriasis after two to three months. (But for 3.6 grams of EPA, you'd need to take about 20 grams of fish oil!) Supplementing with fish oil can also help prevent the increase in blood levels of triglycerides that occurs as a side effect of certain drugs used to treat psoriasis (for example, etretinate and acitretin).

PREGNANCY AND INFANCY

A developing fetus obtains EFAs through the mother's dietary consumption. Omega-3 EFA supplementation has shown many benefits for both the pregnant mother and the developing child, including prolonging gestation and preventing preterm labor. In 2002, in a randomized, double-blind, placebo-controlled study, which is the most stringent way to evaluate an effect, S. F. Olsen and colleagues showed that supplementation with DHA prolonged gestation by six days. In 2003, C. M. Smuts and colleagues showed that supplementation with fish oil prolonged gestation in women at high risk for preterm delivery. In 2000 S. F. Olsen and colleagues showed that women who supplemented with 2.7 grams of fish oil per day showed significantly reduced preterm delivery rates, increased mean birth weight (by 209 grams), and increased duration of pregnancy compared with a control group. These researchers concluded that fish oil's ability to inhibit the production of pro-inflammatory prostaglandins is most likely the mechanism of action.

In 2002 the U.S. Food and Drug Administration (FDA) approved the inclusion of omega-3 and omega-6 EFAs in infant formula. Both types of EFAs are potentially important in infant development, since DHA, EPA, and arachidonic acid are required to make the phospholipid membranes of cells. Supplementation with DHA could be especially important, since this fatty acid is predominant in the membranes of cells in the brain and in the retina of the eyes. A recent study showed visual improvement at four months in infants given omega-3 EFAs in their formula as compared with infants fed nonsupplemented formula. One of the most interesting studies on omega-3 EFA supplementation and infants was done by I. B. Helland and colleagues, as reported in the respected journal *Pediatrics* in 2003. These researchers noted a sustained increase in intelligence and visual acuity at four years of age in children whose mothers were supplemented with fish oil from eighteen weeks of pregnancy to three months postpartum.

Note: As discussed in Chapter 4, in 2004 the FDA issued a warning that set a limit on the amount of fish a pregnant mother should consume due to mercury toxicity concerns for the infant. Therefore, all recommendations for omega-3 EFA supplementation are for fish oil supplements, which are distilled to remove such toxins.

POSTPARTUM DEPRESSION

Mothers are the sole source of nutrients for their babies during development. For this reason mothers can become depleted of many nutrients during pregnancy, especially omega-3 EFAs, which can be harmful for both mother and infant. Several studies now show that mothers can develop postpartum depression when they become depleted of omega-3 EFAs, in particular DHA. Maternal DHA status can be reduced by half during pregnancy and not fully restored for many weeks after delivery, especially if the mother is breast-feeding. An adequate supply of DHA in the mother is necessary to support optimal neurological development of the fetus and infant and is especially important for the development of the infant's synapses (the means by which a nerve cell communicates with other cells).

In 1995 J. R. Hibbeln and N. Salem Jr. showed that DHA or EPA depletion due to pregnancy is associated with major depression. Several investigators have reported lower plasma and erythrocyte concentrations of omega-3 fats among depressed subjects. In 2002 J. R. Hibbeln looked at the DHA content in mothers' milk and seafood consumption in twenty-three countries and confirmed that higher rates of postpartum depression are associated with lower amounts of DHA in breast milk and lower rates of seafood consumption.

Supplementation with EFAs during and after pregnancy is now considered standard in most obstetrical practices in order to provide sufficient amounts of EFAs to both mother and child.

MENSTRUAL PAIN

After ovulation, fatty acids build up in cell membranes in the uterus. After the onset of progesterone withdrawal, before menstruation, these fatty acids are released, causing a concurrent release of a cascade of prostaglandins and leukotrienes. Menstrual pain is associated with increased contractions of smooth muscles in the uterus caused by the autonomic nerve system, hormones, and these locally acting prostaglandins and leukotrienes derived from both omega-6 EFAs (inflammatory) and omega-3 EFAs (anti-inflammatory).

Generally, the omega-6 EFAs produce prostaglandins that increase smooth muscle contractions, whereas prostaglandins derived from omega-3 EFAs do not cause such severe contractions. Susceptible women (especially young women) who eat a typical modern diet that is weighted heavily toward omega-6 EFAs therefore experience increased contractions. These prostaglandins cause not only localized cramps but also nausea and headache. Furthermore, they cause constriction of blood vessels, which may also cause pain. Currently, menstrual pain is treated by preventing ovulation using oral contraceptives and also by inhibiting prostaglandin synthesis with NSAIDs such as aspirin and ibuprofen.

In 1995 a Danish study examined the relationship between intake of omega-3 EFAs and menstrual pain. The researchers evaluated 181 Danish women aged twenty to forty-five years who were not pregnant and were not using oral contraceptives. They found that women with menstrual pain had on average about an 80 percent lower intake of omega-3 EFAs compared to those without pain. The researchers concluded that a high intake of omega-3 EFAs reduces menstrual pain.

A 1996 study evaluated the impact of omega-3 EFA supplementation on menstrual pain. Forty-two girls with menstrual pain were supplemented with 1.8 grams of either a combination of EPA and DHA or a placebo for two months. After two months, the EPA/DHA group reported a significant reduction in menstrual pain and in the use of painkillers, as compared to the placebo group. At the end of the study 70 percent of the girls claimed that they would recommend treatment with omega-3 EFAs for menstrual pain. The researchers also concluded that increasing the amount of dietary omega-3 EFAs, whether by a higher intake of fish or omega-3 EFA supplementation, can provide symptom relief to women with menstrual pain.

ATTENTION-DEFICIT HYPERACTIVITY DISORDER

Attention-deficit hyperactivity disorder (ADHD) is the name of a group of behaviors found in many children and adults. Children with ADHD have trouble paying attention in school and at home and may be much more active and/or impulsive than is usual for their age. These behaviors contribute to significant problems in relationships and learning. ADHD is common, affecting 4 to 12 percent of school-age children. It's more common in boys than in girls.

Because recent generations have seen a rapid rise in the diagnosis of ADHD along with the considerable changes in our diet that we have discussed, many researchers have looked for a dietary cause of this disorder. Studies on children with ADHD have shown that they tend to have lower-than-normal levels of omega-3 EFAs in their red blood cell membranes. A 2000 study by Burgess and colleagues at Purdue University of children with ADHD and dyslexia, a learning disorder often associated with ADHD, found that boys with low blood levels of omega-3 EFAs have a greater tendency to have the problems with behavior, learning, and health consistent with ADHD. Other studies have also indicated that symptoms associated with a deficiency in fatty acids are exhibited to a greater extent in children with ADHD. Those symptoms include thirst, frequent urination, and dry skin and hair. Evidence is accumulating that a deficiency of omega-3 EFAs may be tied to problems of behavior, learning, and health. Other research, however, has not linked all children with ADHD to deficiencies of omega-3 EFAs, but such deficiencies appear to be present for a significant subset of ADHD children.

In 2004 G. S. Young and colleagues looked at fatty acid levels in patients with the adult form of ADHD. This study measured the total blood phospholipid fatty acid concentrations in thirty-five control subjects and thirty-seven adults with ADHD symptoms to determine whether adults with ADHD symptoms had lower levels of essential fatty acids, especially omega-3 EFAs. The adults with ADHD symptoms had, in the phospholipids of their red blood cell membranes, significantly lower levels of total polyunsaturated fatty acids, EPA, and DHA and significantly higher levels of total saturated fatty acids.

Despite the findings of EFA deficiencies in both children and adults with ADHD, it has been difficult for researchers to design and execute a randomized, double-blind, placebo-controlled study (the gold standard for studies) to prove that supplementation with omega-3 EFAs can mitigate the symptoms of ADHD. There are several problems with doing a study such as this. First, how much and what amounts of EFAs should be used? Second, should only those subjects deficient in EFAs and also with ADHD be enrolled? And third, for how long should the supplements be given to subjects in order to find significant symptom improvement?

In 2003 L. Stevens and colleagues completed a randomized, double-blind, placebo-controlled pilot study that evaluated the effects of supplementation with polyunsaturated fatty acids on blood fatty-acid composition and behavior in children with ADHD symptoms. Fifty children were randomized into treatment groups that received daily, for four months, either an olive-oil placebo or a supplement containing 480 mg of DHA, 80 mg of EPA, 40 mg of arachidonic acid, 96 mg of gamma-linolenic acid, and 24 mg of vitamin E. The researchers found that supplementation with the polyunsaturated fatty acids led to a substantial increase in the proportions of EPA, DHA, and vitamin E in the subjects' plasma phospholipids and red blood cell total lipids. For most outcomes, improvement in the group supplemented with polyunsaturated fatty acids was consistently nominally better than that of the olive oil group. Significant improvement was found specifically in conduct problems as rated by parents and attention symptoms as rated by teachers. The supplemented group also showed a decrease in defiant behavior, as compared with the olive-oil group. Also, significant correlations were found between increasing EPA in the red blood cells and decreasing disruptive behavior and improved attention. The researchers concluded that this pilot study suggested the need for further research with both omega-3 EFAs and vitamin E in children with behavioral disorders.

DEVELOPMENTAL COORDINATION DISORDER

Developmental coordination disorder (DCD) affects about 5 percent of school-age children. Those affected show specific difficulties with motor coordination as well as difficulties in learning, behavior, and social or psychological adjustment. This condition usually persists into adulthood. Like ADHD, DCD is also associated with a deficiency of omega-3 EFAs. As we have discussed, these fatty acids are essential for brain development and function.

In a 2005 randomized, double-blind, placebo-controlled trial (the only kind of study that can provide clear evidence of cause and effect), A. J. Richardson and P. Montgomery evaluated 117 children with DCD for three months. Half of them received a supplement containing 80 percent fish oil (omega-3 EFAs) and 20 percent evening primrose oil (omega-6 EFAs). The other half received a placebo. The children were assessed for motor coordination skills, reading and spelling achievement, and teacher ratings of behavior and learning difficulties usually associated with ADHD. After three months of treatment in parallel groups, the changes in motor skills did not differ between the two groups on objective testing. However, children who received the fatty acid supplement showed significantly better progress in both reading and spelling than children who received the placebo. Similarly, active treatment was associated with highly significant reductions in ADHD-related symptoms according to teacher ratings of the children's behavior.

The researchers concluded that the results indicate that fatty acid supplementation may offer a safe and efficacious treatment option for educational and behavioral problems in children with DCD.

AUTISM AND ASPERGER'S SYNDROME

Asperger's syndrome is one of the conditions found on the autism spectrum. The condition involves a number of symptoms, including social problems, vulnerability to sensory overload, awkward posture, and a tendency to take many figures of speech literally. Early research has shown that children with ADHD, autism, and related disorders have been shown to have significantly lower levels of EFAs in their red blood cells. Supplementation with omega-3 and omega-6 EFAs has been considered the next step to a possible dietary treatment for Asperger's in children.

In 2005 L. Patrick and R. Salik evaluated the effects of a fish-oil supplement on language development and learning skills in twenty-two children aged three to ten years who had been diagnosed with autism or Asperger's syndrome and were not currently taking an EFA supplement. The supplement of EFAs included 247 mg of omega-3 EFAs, 40 mg of omega-6 EFAs, and 27 international units (IU) of vitamin E and was given daily for a period of ninety days. Standard assessment tools were used to measure eight primary areas of language and learning, play skills, social interaction, and generalization. The results at the end of the study showed that all children displayed significant increases in their language and learning skills.

Although the etiology as to why developmental disorders such as autism in children have been shown to coincide with low levels of EFAs is unknown, some research suggests that increased oxidative stress in the brain tissue of children with these conditions may lead to increased cellular injury and the need for additional EFAs for cell membrane repair. W. R. McGinnis reported in 2004 that there is greater free-radical production and higher excitotoxic markers, such as glutamate neurotransmitter, in the brains of autistic children. To treat oxidative stress some researchers have used potent antioxidants such as vitamin C, which has been reported to mitigate autistic behavior. McGinnis concluded that benefits from these antioxidants and other nutritional interventions may be due to the reduction of oxidative stress.

ALZHEIMER'S DISEASE

Alzheimer's disease is named after Alois Alzheimer, a German physician who in 1906 discovered abnormal brain tissue in a woman who had died of a mental illness. The abnormal clumps and tangled fiber bundles he found are today referred to as amyloid plaques and neurofibrillary tangles, respectively, and they are symptomatic of Alzheimer's disease. The plaques and tangles are difficult to discern by CT scan or MRI and generally must be seen under a microscope, typically after death. Therefore, an Alzheimer's diagnosis is usually based on symptoms of mental deterioration rather than on physiological changes.

The brain damage of Alzheimer's disease is caused by the protein beta-amyloid, which is toxic to nerve cells. When beta-amyloid levels become excessive, large areas of brain cells are destroyed, resulting in amyloid plaques. The plaques can affect almost any area of the brain and leave deficits in thought control, memory, language, and other mental abilities. There is no cure for Alzheimer's at this time, and treatment of the disease centers on preventing symptoms from worsening once the disease has been diagnosed.

It is believed that as many as 4.5 million Americans have Alzheimer's. The disease usually begins after age sixty. It is the most common form of dementia among the elderly, and risk increases with age, such that symptoms can be found in about 5 percent of men and women ages sixty-five to seventy-four and, as some studies indicate, up to 50 percent of persons older than eighty-five. While younger people also may get Alzheimer's, it is much less common.

Alzheimer's and Omega-3 EFAs

Polyunsaturated fatty acids make up 15 to 30 percent of the dry weight of the brain. Arachidonic acid and DHA constitute 80 to 90 percent of that total; arachidonic acid is about two-thirds of it and DHA is one-third. As we have reviewed, sufficient levels of omega-3 EFAs, and especially DHA, are essential for prenatal brain development and normal maintenance of brain function and vision in adults. DHA deficiencies have been linked to cognitive impairment and Alzheimer's disease. Free radicals can more easily disrupt cell membranes that lack DHA (by way of lipid peroxidation), and indeed, brain-cell membranes of Alzheimer's patients have been found to be deficient in DHA. These DHA deficiencies can be attributed in part to decreased dietary intake of omega-3 EFAs. The deficiencies and the increased oxidative stress can result in brain-cell death.

Dozens of studies have shown a protective effect associated with increased fish consumption and intake of omega-3 EFAs for Alzheimer's patients. The natural conclusion is that diets rich in omega-3 EFAs may be beneficial in reducing the risk for developing Alzheimer's. The exact mechanisms are not completely clear, but much research indicates that Alzheimer's disease is an inflammatory condition, and therefore the ability of omega-3 EFAs to reduce inflammation may be one of the protective factors.

In 2000 W. E. Connor and colleagues reported that feeding animals a diet depleted in omega-3 EFAs limits their learning ability, but learning is restored when they are switched to diets supplemented with DHA. This negative effect of omega-3 depletion on brain function in the absence of neurodegenerative pathology may contribute to an increased risk of Alzheimer's in humans. In 2004 P. K. Mukherjee and colleagues found that DHA was neuroprotective because it reduced beta-amyloid toxicity. In 2002, by giving animals DHA prior to injury, M. Hashimoto and colleagues showed that DHA prevented brain cell death and reduced learning decline. Researchers don't know whether to attribute DHA's beneficial effects to a direct effect on beta-amyloid or to an ability to reduce beta-amyloid production. However, membranes that are rich in DHA seem to have a more protective effect on nerve cells and seem to allow for greater cell fluidity, which allows for the more rapid removal of potentially toxic buildups of proteins that can lead to amyloid proteins.

Inflammation and Alzheimer's Disease

Inflammation also plays a key role in Alzheimer's. When the Alzheimer's plaques appear, the brain reacts to this abnormal tissue via the inflammatory response, which worsens the clinical symptoms as the body's immune response tries to rid itself of this tissue. This fact was initially discovered in a clinical study by W. F. Stewart and colleagues in 1997, who looked at 1,686 participants in the Baltimore Longitudinal Study of Aging and found that the risk of Alzheimer's disease was reduced among users of aspirin and other NSAIDs, whereas the use of acetaminophen, which has no anti-inflammatory activity, did not alter the risk. The researchers concluded that this protection against Alzheimer's suggested that the disease was caused by or worsened due to an inflammatory process. As further evidence, in 2002, R. Schmidt and colleagues evaluated levels of C-reactive protein, an indicator of inflammation, in a twenty-five-year follow-up of the Honolulu-Asia Aging Study. They found that men with the highest levels of C-reactive protein had three times the risk for all dementias, including Alzheimer's disease, compared to men with the lowest levels.

The omega-3 EFA DHA is found in comparatively great concentrations in nerve cell membranes and especially at the synaptic membrane, where cells communicate. Depletion of DHA and an increase in saturated fats in the diet have been demonstrated to effect more aggressive inflammatory responses in the brain cells that surround amyloid plaques, with significant activation of excessive oxidative-stress free radicals and inflammatory cytokines in these areas. DHA supplementation can reduce oxidative stress, as F. Calon and colleagues showed in 2004, and decrease levels of oxidized protein (a measure of the severity of oxidation taking place) by 57 percent.

Some have suggested that supplementation with anti-inflammatories could prevent Alzheimer's disease. Because of the side effects of aspirin and other NSAIDs, which we discussed in Chapter 2, and the fact that this supplementation with anti-inflammatories would need to be long term, it appears that omega-3 EFA supplementation would be preferable, and it has fewer side effects and potentially greater cardiovascular benefits as well.

The Western Diet and Alzheimer's Disease

Because of the growing evidence that some components of Alzheimer's disease are related to the types of fats we eat and their metabolic reactions in the body, there now exists the possibility of intervention with dietary modification, omega-3 EFA supplements, and lipid-lowering agents such as statins. There are two types of Alzheimer's disease. The rarer, early-onset type of Alzheimer's is thought to be a genetic disorder involving abnormalities of amyloid production and metabolism. However, the most common form of Alzheimer's is the late-onset type, which initiates after the age of sixty and has no known genetic links. The latest theory on the development of late-onset Alzheimer's suggests an interaction between some unknown genetic weakness and environmental factors leading to cell death from amyloid toxicity. Persons with late-onset Alzheimer's often have a particular form of the blood protein called apolipoprotein E (apoE): the form of apoE often associated with late-onset Alzheimer's disease is produced by the apoE4 gene. The apoE proteins are known to bind to the beta-amyloid peptide and lead to increased deposition of the toxic amyloid-beta peptide in the brain. People with the disease are about three times more likely to have the apoE4 gene than unaffected controls, but this is not true in every part of the world. Several studies now show that environmental and dietary factors can result in different expressions of the disease. For example, persons in developing countries who carry apoE4 have a lower risk of developing Alzheimer's compared to similar subjects in the West who carry the same apolipoprotein. Further study has shown that the significant difference lies in the amount of saturated fats in the diet. In 2002 Petot and colleagues reported a dramatic increase in the risk of late-onset Alzheimer's in people consuming a very-high-fat diet in their later life. The etiology again is believed to be related to the inflammatory response to the saturated fats and associated oxidative stress on the brain cells.

PARKINSON'S DISEASE

Parkinson's disease is the most common movement disorder and the second most prevalent nerve-destroying disease, after Alzheimer's. Parkinson's is estimated to afflict about 1 million Americans, and about 1 percent of the population over sixty years of age. As the American population ages over the next fifteen to twenty years, the total number of cases is likely to double. All races and ethnic groups are affected. Parkinson's disease is associated with progressive disability and often increased mortality. It is caused by disruption of the neurotransmitter dopamine, which is made by brain cells in the basal ganglia. Treatments for this condition generally are drugs that can either provide dopamine or cause dopamine to stay in the brain cells longer.

In 2005 de Lau and colleagues evaluated more than 5,000 people older than fifty-five to determine the association between consumption of polyunsaturated fatty acids and the risk of developing Parkinson's. After an average follow-up of six years, fifty-one participants developed Parkinson's. The members of this group were found to have significantly fewer polyunsaturated fatty acids in their diet as compared to the norms. The authors concluded that a higher intake of polyunsaturated fatty acids, like the omega-3 EFAs found in fish oils, might protect against Parkinson's disease.

DEPRESSION

Clinical depression is characterized by the persistent incidence of sadness, inappropriate crying, and feelings of worthlessness or hopelessness. Any persistent depressive symptoms need prompt medical investigation by a medical professional. Depressive symptoms may also indicate some type of underlying physiological disorder. Various related depression-like physical symptoms (including fatigue, lethargy, and weakness) could be symptoms of an underlying condition such as chronic fatigue syndrome, diabetes, fibromyalgia, or Parkinson's disease.

Research has now shown that symptoms of depression are more common in those who consume lesser amounts of omega-3 EFAs, which has led to a new area of treatments for depression. Several studies have reported depletions of omega-3 fats among depressed patients, and a cross-national comparison has revealed a significant inverse correlation between annual prevalence of major depression and fish consumption. In 2001 A. Tanskanen evaluated 3,204 Finnish adults and evaluated depressive symptoms along with measuring their fish consumption and found the likelihood of having depressive symptoms was significantly higher among infrequent fish consumers than among frequent consumers. Additionally, in 1998, M. Peet and colleagues found that depressed patients have depleted levels of plasma and cell membrane omega-3 EFAs and particularly of DHA.

Fish contains high concentrations of omega-3 polyunsaturated fatty acids. Both EPA and DHA are found in fish oil, and DHA in particular is believed to be required for optimal neuronal (brain cell) function. A reduction in our dietary intake of fish may predispose us to depressive illnesses. Reports on our ancient Paleolithic ancestors indicate that human beings evolved consuming diets containing approximately equivalent proportions of omega-3 and omega-6 fatty acids, a balance that may be considered optimal for brain development and function. As we have learned, corn-, soy-, and other vegetable-based oils, which are rich in omega-6 fats, were not available in abundance during much of human evolution but now dominate the modern Western diet. In fact, over the past 100 years or so we have lowered the ratio of omega-3 to omega-6 EFAs in our diet to possibly as high as 1 to 25. Correspondingly, during the past century, the prevalence of major depression has increased worldwide.

There is now evidence that major depression is accompanied by an acute phase response in which there is an increase in the production of pro-inflammatory prostaglandins, cytokines, and leukotrienes. A dietary imbalance of omega-6 and omega-3 fatty acids can also result in an overproduction of these pro-inflammatory factors. Rebalancing the inflammatory state may help mitigate symptoms in patients experiencing depression, as clinical studies of omega-3 EFA supplementation have shown. In 2002 M. Peet and D. F. Horrobin reported on the addition of a daily dose of 1, 2, or 4 grams of EPA or a placebo to the treatment of patients who had failed to respond to initial antidepressant medication. The EPA groups had a marked improvement relative to those on placebo. The improvement was dose-dependent, with the 1-gram dose producing the biggest improvement and the larger dosages having progressively less effect. In 2002 B. Nemets and colleagues added ethyl-EPA or placebo to maintenance antidepressant therapy in a group of patients with a major depressive disorder uncontrolled by medication. They found highly significant benefits from the addition of EPA compared with placebo by the end of the third week of treatment. Interestingly, despite depressed patients' brains having been found to have lower levels of DHA than EPA, in 2000 L. B. Marangell found no beneficial effects of supplementing depressed patients with DHA alone, which is believed to have a lesser anti-inflammatory effect.

Furthermore, it has been discovered that the inflammatory cytokines, especially tumor necrosis factor alpha, activated in depression can affect the hypothalamic adrenal axis, inducing resistance to the effects of the body's own powerful anti-inflammatory steroid (glucocorticoid) hormones. The depressive state can result, therefore, in the inflammatory factors of the body going unchecked, which consequentially depletes omega-3 EFA stores.

In addition, the increase in the omega-6 content of the Western diet, at the cost of omega-3 EFAs, most likely contributes to an increased incidence of cardiovascular disease and inflammatory disorders, as we discussed earlier in this chapter, and these conditions, along with lower levels of HDL cholesterol, are related to depression.

Finally, an interesting report by J. R. Hibbeln in 2002 noted that the DHA content of mothers' milk (which reflects the maternal omega-3 EFA status) and mothers' seafood consumption both predict prevalence rates of postpartum depression. That is, the lower the content of DHA in breast milk, and the lower the mother's consumption of seafood, the greater the likelihood of the mother developing postpartum depression.

BIPOLAR DISORDER

Bipolar disorder, sometimes referred to as manic-depressive illness, is a common psychiatric illness associated with high morbidity and early death. The disease involves overactive cell signal transduction. Signal transduction at the cellular level refers to the movement of signals from outside the cell to inside it. The eventual outcome is an alteration in cellular activity and changes in the program of genes expressed within the cell. Supplementation with omega-3 EFAs can inhibit signal transduction mechanisms in brain cell membranes, and high-dose omega-3 EFAs can be effective mood stabilizers in bipolar disorder. In 1999 A. L. Stoll and colleagues conducted a double-blind, placebo-controlled trial involving thirty patients with bipolar disorder and found that omega-3 supplements along with standard treatment had a significant beneficial effect in mitigating symptoms.

SCHIZOPHRENIA

Schizophrenia is one of the most disabling of all psychiatric illnesses. Pharmacologic treatments for the disease often leave schizophrenia patients with residual symptoms, lethargy, and cognitive impairment.

D. F. Horrobin, a renowned expert in schizophrenia, has proposed a "membrane phospholipid" model of schizophrenia. The model states that the metabolism of an abnormal composition of phospholipids in brain cells is responsible for the range of symptoms that are classified as schizophrenia. According to Horrobin's theory, decreased levels of EFAs result in less DHA and EPA for the brain to incorporate into nerve cell membranes, and this deficiency results in abnormal phospholipid composition and therefore abnormal function of the membrane-based neurotransmitter systems. In this model, omega-3 EFA supplementation has the potential to normalize the composition of phospholipids in the brain, preventing dysfunction of the dopaminergic and serotonergic neurotransmitter receptors.

Various studies have shown benefits of omega-3 EFA supplementation in patients with chronic schizophrenia who were not being treated concurrently with conventional antipsychotic medications. Other studies have indicated a reduction in the severity of symptoms ranging from 17 to 85 percent when 1 to 2 grams per day of omega-3 EFAs were added to patients' usual antipsychotic medications. Similar studies with schizophrenic patients on antipsychotic medications have not shown similar benefits with supplementation of 3 grams per day of omega-3 EFAs. Researchers have concluded that the best results for treating schizophrenia can be achieved at a dose of 2 grams per day, which produces in red blood cells an increase in EPA without any decrease in arachidonic acid. At higher dosages, researchers have postulated, the increase in red blood cell EPA is accompanied by a substantial decrease in arachidonic acid, a fatty acid that plays a central role in many neuronal signal transduction systems.

CANCER PROTECTION

Research has demonstrated that cancer is a largely avoidable disease. It is estimated that more than two-thirds of cancer may be prevented through lifestyle modification. Nearly one-third of cancer occurrences can be attributed to diet alone. The typical American diet that is high in fat, low in fiber, and lacking fruit and vegetables has been consistently shown to increase the risk of many cancers. But while studies have shown that a lack of omega-3 EFAs in the diet can contribute to cancer risk, they also have shown that supplementing with omega-3 EFAs may help prevent it.

Prostate Cancer

Population studies show that Asian men living in Asia have a 2 percent lifetime risk of prostate cancer; when they move to North America, the risk in the next generation jumps to 10 percent. One possible reason is the typically fatty Western diet. A number of studies have shown that men who eat a low-fiber, high-fat diet have a higher rate of prostate cancer than those who eat a high-fiber, low-fat diet, and that foods rich in saturated fats are associated with increased risk of prostate cancer development, possibly because those fats are metabolized into testosterone. Omega-3 EFAs may be protective against prostate cancer. In 2001 P. Terry and colleagues published a study of more than 6,000 Swedish men that the researchers had followed from age fifty-five for thirty years to see whether eating fatty fish would reduce the risk of prostate cancer. During the thirty years, 466 men were diagnosed with prostate cancer, and 340 of these men died. The men who ate no fish had a twofold to threefold higher risk of prostate cancer than those who ate moderate or high amounts. Other studies found that omega-3 EFAs can inhibit the growth of prostate cancer cells in the laboratory dish and in animals, and still others found that the higher the concentration of fatty acids in a man's bloodstream, the lower his risk of prostate cancer. Researchers have concluded that fatty-fish consumption lowers the risk of prostate cancer through inhibition of arachidonic-acid-derived eicosanoid biosynthesis, since EPA competes with arachidonic acid for the cyclooxygenase enzyme in order to be converted to the anti-inflammatory eicosanoids. And higher concentrations of EPA can lead to important changes in relative concentrations of tumor-growth-enhancing prostaglandins, resulting in a reduced risk of prostate cancer.

Breast Cancer

A. Tsubura and colleagues in 2005 concluded that multiple factors contribute to the development of human breast cancer, but dietary factors most likely have the greatest effects. Based on their research, the dietary component most strongly associated with the development of breast cancer is saturated fat. In contrast, a diet high in omega-3 EFAs and low in omega-6 EFAs is protective against breast cancer.

In another study on breast cancer, V. Pala and colleagues in 2001 evaluated 4,052 postmenopausal women for five and a half years. Of these women, seventy-one developed invasive breast cancer. Women with highest DHA concentrations had less than half the risk of breast cancer of women with the lowest amounts. Interestingly, a higher concentration of monounsaturated fats, especially oleic acid, in their body tissue was associated with a significantly increased risk. Oleic acid is a fatty acid found in animal and vegetable oils used to make synthetic butters and cheeses. It is also used to flavor baked goods, candy, ice cream, and sodas. The researchers pointed out that most oleic acid in mammalian tissue is derived from saturated stearic acid through a process involving the enzyme delta-9-desaturase. Saturated fatty acids, cholesterol, carbohydrates, insulin, testosterone, and estrogen all activate this enzyme, whereas dietary polyunsaturated fatty acids, such as those found in fish oil, and fasting can deactivate it.

Colorectal Cancer

Colorectal cancer was responsible for about 56,000 deaths in the United States in 2004. The American Cancer Society estimates that about 130,000 new cases of colorectal cancer are diagnosed every year. A link has now been established between the development of colon cancer and elevation of levels of CRP, a marker of inflammation circulating in the blood that, as we discussed earlier, is associated with an increased risk of heart disease. In 2004 T. P. Erlinger published the results of a study of 22,000 adults showing that people with high blood levels of CRP were more likely to develop colorectal cancers than those with low levels of CRP. The study also found that the odds of developing colorectal cancers increased progressively with higher concentrations of CRP. Overall, people whose CRP levels were in the highest 25 percent had twice the risk of developing colorectal cancer and 2.5 times the risk of developing colon cancer as those whose levels were in the lowest 25 percent. Among nonsmokers, those whose CRP levels were in the highest 25 percent were 2.5 times as likely to develop colorectal cancer and 3.5 times as likely to develop colon cancer as those whose levels were in the lowest 25 percent. Those who had taken either aspirin or an NSAID agent within the forty-eight hours prior to the blood draw had a CRP level indicating a reduced risk of colorectal cancer. Based on this link to inflammation, much of the preventive colon cancer research had been with NSAIDs, but after the very public negative cardiac results of the VIGOR study (discussed in Chapter 2), many began to reconsider omega-3 EFAs and whether their anti-inflammatory effects could prevent colon cancer.

In 1992 M. Anti and colleagues evaluated the effects of twelve weeks of omega-3 EFA supplementation on twenty patients with sporadic adenomatous colorectal polyps, a form of premalignant colon polyps. The treatment group of ten received a daily fish-oil supplement containing 4.1 grams of EPA and 3.6 grams of DHA; the other ten subjects received a placebo. After two weeks of treatment subjects in the fish oil group showed fewer cellular changes indicative of cancer compared to the placebo group. The EPA content in rectal mucosa increased in the fish oil group, and arachidonic acid levels decreased. The fish-oil-induced cellular changes of the polyps were related to omega-3 EFA effects on the arachidonic-acid-derived prostaglandin pathway. The authors of this study concluded that fish oil exerts a rapid effect that may protect high-risk subjects from colon cancer.

In 2004, B. Reddy published a review of ninety-one studies on the relationship between diet and cancer, providing substantial evidence that diets rich in the omega-3 fats found in cold-water fish help prevent colon cancer. The review included studies conducted in the United States, Canada, and twenty-two European countries that show that the tumor-promoting effect seen with dietary fat depends on which type of fat it is, and that colon cancer risk is related more to what type of fat, rather than how much fat, is eaten. Although the ways in which omega-3 fats exert their protective effects is not yet fully understood, it appears that the fats a person eats affect the amount of bile acids he or she excretes. People eating a typical Western diet, which is high in saturated and omega-6 fats, who are at higher risk of colon cancer, also excrete high levels of bile acids. Excess bile acids have been shown to stimulate an inflammatory chemical called protein kinase C, to induce cell proliferation, and to act as promoters in colon carcinogenesis. Omega-3 fats are thought to prevent carcinogen activation by decreasing DNA damage, enhancing DNA repair, and enhancing apoptosis (programmed cell death) in carcinogenic colonic cells.

Chemotherapy

Fish oils, either taken as a supplement or eaten in fish, have also demonstrated beneficial effects for patients receiving chemotherapy for cancer. Most dramatically, researchers have found that they can significantly slow the rate of weight loss associated with most forms of chemotherapy and stabilize adipose tissue and muscle mass. The general physical wasting commonly seen in cancer patients is called cachexia, and it results not only from the disease but from the toxic chemotherapies used to treat it. Cachexia often is associated with weakness, fatigue, and poor quality of life and can result in depression, poor outcome, and greater morbidity. Cachexia is thought to be caused by the release of inflammatory cytokines and other factors secreted by the tumor, such as tumor necrosis factor-alpha (TNF-α), interleukin-1ß, interleukin-6, and proteolysis-inducing factor, which can break down protein and result in muscle tissue. Good nutrition, caloric supplementation, and hydration are critical when treating cancer. EPA (concentrated in fish oil supplements) at doses ranging from 1 to 6 grams per day has been shown to result in weight stabilization after three to four weeks and 1 to 2 kilograms of weight gain after seven weeks in cancer patients. Animal studies suggest that EPA works by suppressing the effect of proteolysis-inducing factor along with suppressing the inflammatory cytokines.

Essential fatty acids themselves have been shown to be cytotoxic to a variety of tumor cells in vitro. In 1997 M. Iigo and colleagues found in a Japanese population that DHA can exert marked antimetastatic activity on lung tumor cells. They also found that DHA effects a pronounced change in the membrane characteristics of tumor cells, such that uptake of DHA into tumor cells results in a decrease in the cells' ability to metastasize.

Drug resistance in tumor cells is a major problem in chemotherapy. U. N. Das and colleagues reported in 1998 that gamma-linolenic acid (omega-6) and EPA (omega-3) can increase the effectiveness of many anticancer drugs on human cervical carcinoma cells in vitro. Alpha-linolenic acid, gamma-linolenic acid, EPA, and DHA all showed an ability to enhance the uptake of chemotherapy drugs in these cancer cells. In addition, DHA, EPA, gamma-linolenic acid, and dihomo-gamma-linolenic acid were found to be toxic to some degree to the human cervical carcinoma cells in the lab.

CHAPTER 6

Fish Oil Supplements: Finding a Good-Quality Product and the Appropriate Dosage

Fish oil is hot!

Approximately 35 percent of adults take dietary supplements on a daily basis. The fish oil supplements industry in particular has seen phenomenal growth in recent times, at a rate of about 50 percent per year. In 2003 consumers in the United States spent $190 million on fish oil supplements, and that amount is predicted to have increased to $310 million in 2005. Not all fish oil supplements are the same, however, due to the types of fish the oil is extracted from, the processing techniques, and the storage conditions. As is the case with most consumer items, you generally get what you pay for. The major manufacturing concerns that separate high-quality supplements from the rest of the pack are purity, potency, and oxidation, each of which we will discuss, followed by some general guidelines for dosages.

PURITY

As we discussed in Chapter 4, it is important to limit the amount of fresh fish in our regular diet because fish can store and concentrate in their flesh heavy metals (mercury and lead) and other toxins, such as polychlorinated biphenyls (PCBs). This same caution applies to fish oil supplements if special purification techniques are not used in the manufacturing process. Fortunately, many manufacturing techinques have been found to remove these potentially deadly toxins from fish oil. In 2004 ConsumerLab.com, a product-claims watchdog group, evaluated forty-one different fish oil supplements and found no detectable levels of mercury or other toxins in them. This is good news for the industry, as the supplements that were tested included both high- and low-end fish oil products.

The purification technique most commonly used by manufacturers is molecular distillation. This process, which takes place in a vacuum, uses very low heat and enzymes to remove heavy metals, certain vitamins, and saturated fats, leaving behind the omega-3 essential fatty acids (EFAs).

Why, you might ask, are vitamins removed? The fat-soluble vitamins A and D are removed due to their high concentrations in natural fish oil. Unlike water-soluble vitamins, which are excreted in the urine and stored in the body only to a limited extent, fat-soluble vitamins are stored in body fat and can cause toxicity when taken in excess amounts. The recommended daily allowance for vitamin A is 5,000 international units (IU) for adults and 8,000 IU for pregnant or lactating women. The recommended daily allowance for vitamin D is 200 IU, but recently, studies now suggest to increase it to 400–800 IU per day.

POTENCY

What is the difference between low-end and high-end fish oil supplements? Generally, the difference is the amount and type of EPA and docosahexaenoic acid (DHA) they contain.

EPA and DHA Concentrations

Most high-end, more expensive fish oil supplements have considerably higher potencies of EPA and DHA per capsule. The majority of studies we reviewed in Chapter 5 employed dosages in the range of 2 to 4 grams of EPA/DHA. A lower-end 1-gram fish oil capsule typically provides only 180 milligrams (mg) of EPA and 120 mg of DHA; the rest of the capsule content is "marine product," a mix

---

THIRD-PARTY VERIFICATION

Manufacturers of higher-quality fish oil products often contract with a third-party laboratory to assess purity and label accuracy, and they will often post the lab's documentation on their Web site or publish other advertisements. Many companies also claim that their fish oil is "pharmaceutical grade." Such a claim might lead you to assume that there is a certifying agency that validates the quality of fish oils. In fact, there is no such agency. In most cases the term *pharmaceutical grade* means that a fish oil supplement has the highest level of purity and potency such a product can have: its ingredients are over 99 percent pure, with no binders, fillers, dyes, or unknown substances, and it has superior concentrations of potent EPA and DHA. This standard could be considered analogous to similar high-quality standards that pharmaceutical companies must adhere to. However, buyer beware, because currently in the United States there is no regulated definition of "pharmaceutical-grade" fish oil.

of many different fatty acids and cholesterol with very few omega-3 EFAs. In order to achieve a potent dosage of, say, 3 grams with this product, we would need to take ten capsules per day. This amount of oil can often cause burping, loose stools, and at the very least fishy breath.

In contrast, higher-end fish oil capsules typically provide 600 to 850 mg of EPA/DHA per capsule. In order to achieve a dosage of 3 grams with this type of product, we would need to take only four or five capsules per day. Fish oil is also available as a concentrated liquid that provides 1 to 3 grams of EPA/DHA per teaspoon. At this low volume, any fishy aftertaste and bloating would most likely stop after about one week.

The best way to determine the quantity of omega-3 EFAs that a fish oil supplement contains is to look on the product label for the nutritional breakdown and serving amount. Higher-quality fish oil supplements will cost more, because their manufacturers have put them through more processing to concentrate EPA and DHA in them, but you will be able to take fewer of these supplements in order to obtain adequate amounts of omega-3 EFAs.

Ethyl Esters versus Triglycerides

Triglycerides are lipid (fat) molecules comprising a glycerol backbone to which three fatty acids are attached (see Figure 3.1 on page 34). Most fatty acids in the body, including EPA and DHA, are found in triglyceride form. Because EPA/DHA are known to be the desired fatty acids in fish oil, they are often extracted separately and concentrated prior to being added to a fish oil supplement. In the process of being extracted, EPA and DHA are broken out as the ethyl ester form, meaning that they exist as individual fatty acid strands, not as part of the natural triglyceride form.

The natural triglyceride form is superior to the synthetic ethyl ester form in many ways. EPA and DHA ethyl esters are highly unstable and rapidly break down during storage. Also, the ethyl ester form has been shown to be ten to fifty times more resistant to enzymatic digestion than the triglyceride form, and therefore less well absorbed. In fact, the body absorbs the natural triglyceride form up to 300 percent better than the synthetic ester form. Additionally, when fish oils are digested their lipid content is converted into free (single-strand) fatty acids. After being absorbed through the epithelial cells, these free fatty acids are immediately converted into triglycerides. If a glycerol backbone is not available (as would be the case with ethyl esters), and the body has no other glycerol backbones to spare, the fatty acid cannot be converted to triglyceride form. Fatty acids not converted to triglycerides pose an oxidation burden in the form of free radical formation.

In order to stabilize the omega-3 EFAs in their products and maximize the body's absorption of them, manufacturers of high-end fish oil supplements re-triglyceride the ethyl ester forms of extracted, concentrated EPA and DHA. This process is an expensive but important step that at the moment is practiced only by the very top manufacturers (although many other manufacturers are now getting into the act as well). In Sweden, Denmark, Norway, and the UK, only fish oil with EPA and DHA in triglyceride form can be sold due to the stability and absorption issues.

OXIDATION CONCERNS

Fish oil has had a bad reputation among many people who were forced to take cod liver oil as children. Cod liver, high in omega-3 EFAs and vitamins A and D, has been used for more than 200 years to promote good health, but at a price. Its foul smell and taste made an indelible mark on many and left many people resistant to taking the fish oil supplements produced today by modern techniques. The smell and taste problem with cod liver oil is due to rancidity, which is caused by oxidation. Rancidity is a problem for all polyunsaturated fatty acids, including fish, safflower, sunflower seed, flaxseed, and hempseed oils. Polyunsaturated oils can become rancid when exposed to heat, light, or oxygen. Typically, the cod liver oil of yesteryear was exposed to one of these factors during manufacture, storage, and/or sale.

The chemical reaction that results in rancidity is called lipid oxidation. Generally, the more double bonds present in an unsaturated fatty acid, the more readily it oxidizes. Lipid oxidation is a series of reactions between oxygen and the hydrocarbon chains of unsaturated fatty acids. These reactions result in the formation of hydroperoxides and free radicals. These compounds, in turn, react with the remaining fatty acids to produce more hydroperoxides and free radicals, and the process continues. The hydroperoxide reactions create, among others, volatile compounds that are responsible for the foul smell and taste associated with rancidity.

Why Worry about Lipid Oxidation in Fish Oils?

The issue of rancidity in fish oil is not just that it creates a bad sensation for the tongue and nose but that lipid free-radical hydroperoxides, sometimes referred to as peroxides, have been linked to very serious diseases.

Peroxides have been fingered as one of the causes of atherosclerosis, or the development of plaques in blood vessels, which can lead to stroke, aneurysm, and heart attack. The potential presence of lipid peroxides in plaques from human aortas was first noted as early as 1970 by Smith and Van Lier. These authors isolated peroxidation products of cholesterol, another lipid, in plaques taken from the arteries of rabbits. They concluded that eating cholesterol-containing foods could cause cholesterol peroxides to be absorbed and enter the cholesterol pool of the body, and consequently to form plaque deposits. This research, along with some other early investigations on cholesterol in humans, started the whole field of study that has led to the recommendations for a low-cholesterol diet and the development of statin drugs to lower cholesterol.

In 1985 E. Giani and colleagues investigated the effects of consumption of polyunsaturated oils that had been subjected to repeated frying on the production of eicosanoids and prostaglandins and found that rats fed this diet had higher levels of the prostaglandin thromboxane A_2, which can stimulate platelet aggregation and lead to plaque formation and atherosclerosis. They concluded that if rancid polyunsaturated fatty acids are consumed, the oxidative deterioration may promote rather than hinder the progression of atherosclerosis. Therefore, the potential health benefits from consumption of polyunsaturated fatty acids could be negated by lipid peroxidation.

Another disease in which oxidized lipids may play a role is cancer. High-fat diets have been demonstrated to promote the development of cancerous tumors. For example, in 1971 K. K. Carroll and H. T. Khor noted an increased incidence of mammary (breast) tumors associated with high level of peroxides resulting from increased unsaturation of fats in the diet. They concluded that it is possible that the incidence of breast cancer might be lowered by decreasing the amount of fat in the diet. This has been a general recommendation for the prevention of almost all forms of cancer, including those linked to lipid peroxides and other free radicals. The mechanisms in cancer are unclear, but it is thought to be linked to DNA mutations, and evidence shows that dietary interventions such as calorie restriction can decrease the incidence of this disease.

Preventing Lipid Oxidation

Some manufacturers offer flavored fish oil capsules to mask the smell and taste of oxidation. Others offer enteric fish oil capsules, which are coated with a substance that does not dissolve until it has passed through the stomach and entered the small intestines, so that potentially rancid fish oil will not be burped up. However, given that free-radical lipid hydroperoxides have been linked to very serious disease conditions, our focus should be on preventing oxidation, not disguising its symptoms. High-end manufacturers have found that processing fish oil in an oxygen-free environment (usually a nitrogen environment) significantly reduces the oxidative process. Additionally, to prevent the harmful effects associated with free-radical toxicity from lipid hydroperoxides, and to avoid the development of rancidity, most fish oil supplements contain small amounts of antioxidants. Antioxidants have the ability to minimize oxidation and counteract free radicals that can damage cell membranes. Vitamin E is the most common antioxidant additive; lecithin and ascorbyl palmitate are also common. The label of fish oils will have this information and can be useful in determining which type and the amount of an antioxidant is used; the label also contains an expiration date.

High-end manufacturers often measure oxidation levels in their products, and they publish these results on their websites or in promotional literature. Several independent watchdog groups also test oxidation levels in fish oils from various manufacturers. The most common chemical assessments of an oil's oxidation are provided in terms of peroxide value (PV), anisidine value (AV), and totox value. These results generally are given on the manufacturer's website or in the promotional literature. The PV is an assessment of an oil's hydroperoxide content, in units of millimole of hydroperoxide per kilogram of oil. Hydroperoxides decompose into carbonyls and other compounds. This decomposition accelerates as the temperature is raised, so that the PV of an oil may be reduced or eliminated by heating the oil in the absence of oxygen. This is done as part of the refinement process. As a result of this refinement, however, a lower level of natural antioxidants is present in the oil, and the carbonyl compounds now in the oil may further oxidation, resulting in bad taste. The anisidine assay measures these bad-tasting carbonyl compounds; the AV is a better indication of the freshness of an oil. The totox assay measures a different carbonyl present in a processed oil that may also influence taste.

Preventing Oxidation at Home

The fact is that omega-3 EFAs are very good for us, as we have reviewed in this book, but care must be taken with the manufacturing and storage of these oils in order to reduce the amount of lipid oxidation and the associated dangers of consuming a product that has become rancid. Therefore, it may be necessary to spend a few extra dollars on a high-quality fish oil product that uses antioxidants, such as vitamin E, and proper manufacturing with low heat in a nitrogen environment to help ensure a safe and effective product.

At home, fish oil capsules should be stored in a cool, dry place away from direct sunlight. Refrigeration is recommended for liquid fish oil but generally is not necessary for soft gel capsules. These efforts will help prevent oxidation. The surest sign of rancidity is a strong fishy odor, which indicates that the product probably has some oxidation occurring and the oil may be becoming rancid. It is the experience of the authors that high-end fish oils are odor free and therefore are less likely to have oxidized.

The prevention of lipid peroxidation during the cooking of polyunsaturated fats is also important. Polyunsaturated cooking oils, such as canola and safflower oils, should be kept either in the refrigerator or in a dark, cool place to

reduce oxidation. Cooking these oils over high heat can release the toxic peroxides mentioned above, and therefore it is preferable to cook with these oils only
over low heat or to use them without heating, such as for salad dressings. These
cooking oils also have a limited shelf life; purchase them in small quantities and
replace them every few months.

DOSAGES

There are no hard and fast guidelines concerning the optimal amount of omega-
3 EFAs to be consumed. For healthy adults, the World Health Organization recommends 300 to 500 mg of omega-3 EFAs per day, while the National Institutes
of Health recommends 650 mg per day and the American Heart Association recommends 650 to 1,000 mg per day.

The typical Western diet includes a total of about 1.6 grams of EFAs on a
daily basis, of which about 1.4 grams comes from omega-6 EFAs (primarily
linolenic acid) and only about 0.1 to 0.2 grams from omega-3 EFAs. Increasing
our consumption of foods rich in omega-3 EFAs in order to have a more balanced EFA ratio and achieve even the lowest recommended omega-3 dosage is
very difficult. As we discussed in Chapter 4, the best source of omega-3 EFAs in
the diet is fish, but regular consumption of fish carries a potential load of toxins
that can negatively affect the body. And due to the inconsistent or unknown
amounts of omega-3 EFAs in food, it is almost impossible to determine how
much one is actually consuming.

Perhaps the optimal way to assess the best dosage for any individual is to
actually measure the levels of EFAs in the blood through laboratory tests. Barry
Sears, author of *The Zone,* has popularized the arachidonic acid/EPA ratio. By
measuring our blood levels of arachidonic acid, which is the precursor of the
"bad" inflammatory eicosanoids, and EPA, which is the precursor of the "good"
eicosanoids, we can determine the balance of these agents in the body and then
appropriately modify the diet to reduce the arachidonic acid content and increase our supplement intake to raise the EPA content. Sears emphasizes that the
arachidonic acid/EPA ratio in the average American is approximately 11 to 1,
whereas a much, much lower ratio of 1.5 to 3 indicates that the good and bad
eicosanoids are in balance and the body is in the healthiest wellness zone. Most
physicians are not aware of this test, and it can be difficult to get insurers to pay
for it. You can, however, order such a test from a mail-order lab, which will send
you a kit that you can use to obtain your own blood. You can then send the
blood to the lab and have the results mailed directly to you.

In 2003 W. Harris and his associates developed the omega-3 index, which is
a measurement of EPA and DHA levels in red blood cells that indicates adequate
or inadequate levels of omega-3 EFAs in the body. They then further studied

cardiac risk based on these levels and developed a risk assessment for coronary artery disease based on the omega-3 index. In the index, a low level of EPA and DHA levels is a very sensitive marker of increased risk for coronary artery disease and complications. This test is performed with a simple finger stick. Once existing levels of omega-3 EFAs have been determined, the dose of fish oil supplements can be more accurately titrated to achieve healthy levels.

In the absence of specific blood tests we start our patients on 2.5 grams of EPA/DHA per day, broken up into two daily doses, each taken with a meal. We recommend a high-quality fish oil supplement that can provide approximately 1 gram (1,000 mg) of EPA and DHA per capsule; this concentration is higher than that found in many fish oil capsules (which usually have 120 mg of EPA and 180 mg of DHA). Look for the highest concentration possible in order to minimize the number of capsules you need to take.

Dosing for Specific Health Conditions

If you have a significant medical condition you should use these recommendations only as general guidelines. Please check with your personal physician to tailor any dosage to your individual requirements. Your physician should make the final recommendation as to whether you should use fish oil supplements and at what dose. Your personal physician is aware of the many complexities of your condition or disease and should be able to advise you appropriately. General statements such as "You don't need that stuff" or "Since the FDA hasn't approved it, I can't recommend it" should not be accepted as valid in the face of more than 900 clinical trials showing the efficacy of omega-3 EFAs.

Coronary Heart Disease

A relatively low dose of omega-3 fatty acids, at approximately 1 gram per day of EPA/DHA, has been used in most cardiac studies and has been shown to result in significant reductions in the incidence of the risk of nonfatal heart attack, fatal heart attack, sudden death caused by cardiac arrhythmia, and all-cause mortality (death) in patients with known coronary heart disease.

Elevated Triglycerides

Generally, higher dosages of omega-3 fatty acids (2 to 4 grams per day) have been used in studies that show their effectiveness in lowering triglyceride levels in patients with hypertriglyceridemia (elevated blood triglycerides). A dose-related response has been found, such that the higher the triglyceride level is, the higher the dose of omega-3 EFAs that is required. Statins and other cholesterol-lowering drugs do not interfere with the action of omega-3 EFAs, and often both are used in the initial treatment or in the case of very high triglyceride levels.

Some studies have shown an increase in low-density lipoproteins (LDLs, "bad" cholesterol) resulting from high-dose fish oil therapy in patients with abnormal blood lipids, but no significant increase in plaque formation or cardiac events.

Elevated Blood Pressure

Studies on the effects of omega-3 EFAs on patients with hypertension have generally used at least 3 grams of EPA/DHA per day. Most studies indicate a dose-related response, such that the higher the blood pressure, the larger the omega-3 EFA dose required to lower it. Most if not all current blood pressure medications can be taken in conjunction with omega-3 EFA supplements, but as always, the physician who is treating you should make the final recommendation as to whether to use fish oil supplements and at what dose.

Rheumatoid Arthritis

The clinical trials on omega-3 EFAs and rheumatoid arthritis generally have used a dose range between 2 and 6 grams of EPA/DHA daily. As we reviewed in the Chapter 5, arthritis is by definition an inflammatory process. EPA, because it is the major precursor to the anti-inflammatory eicosanoids, is the omega-3 EFA most studied when evaluating this severe form of arthritis, which is also considered an autoimmune disease. Therefore, preparations of EPA and DHA used for inflammatory conditions, such as arthritis, other autoimmune diseases, and vascular inflammation associated with coronary heart disease and stroke, should have a higher ratio of EPA to DHA.

Protection from Cyclosporine Toxicity in Organ Transplant Patients

Several studies have shown a positive kidney-protective effect from using omega-3 EFAs in transplant patients who are on the anti-rejection drug cyclosporine. Nephrotoxicity, or kidney toxicity, is the main serious side effect of cyclosporine treatment. In 1995 S. Badalamenti and colleagues reported that both experimental and clinical data showed that dietary supplementation with fish oil lessens cyclosporine nephrotoxicity, possibly by lowering renal thromboxane (Tx) production. In the study, twenty-six liver transplant patients were divided into two groups, one receiving a fish oil supplement and the other receiving a placebo corn oil supplement. At the end of two months, in the fish oil group the effective renal plasma flow increased by 22 percent, the glomerular filtration rate increased by 33 percent, renal blood flow increased by 17 percent, and renal vascular resistances decreased by 20 percent. No improvements were seen in the patients on corn oil.

The studies done in this area have used very high doses of omega-3 EFAs

(6 to 12 grams per day for up to one year). Anyone who has had a transplant and is on cyclosporine should discuss the use of omega-3 EFA supplementation with their transplant specialist. We cannot fully endorse the use of omega-3 EFA for this condition as a general statement because of the seriousness of this condition and the lack of large-scale studies.

EFA Supplementation during Pregnancy

During pregnancy, EFAs are used by the fetus for the production of prosta-glandins and as structural elements of cell membranes. Therefore, throughout gestation, the mother's EFA requirements markedly increase, especially for DHA, which is the predominant EFA in nervous-system tissue. Effective dosing during pregnancy has been shown to be on average 1 gram of approximately equal parts of EPA and DHA. Data shows that effective maternal supplementation requires a mixture of omega-6 and omega-3 fatty acids, so omega-3 EFAs are generally combined with omega-6 EFAs for pregnancy supplementation.

In one interesting study on omega-3 EFA supplementation during pregnancy and for later childhood allergies, in April 2003, S. L. Prescott reported that women who use fish oil supplements can expect their child to have a reduced risk of developing allergies later in life. The study was conducted in families prone to allergic reactions to eggs, peanuts, pet hair, and dust mites. The babies of moth-ers who took a daily fish oil supplement were three times less likely to develop food allergies and had less severe infant eczema in the first year of life. This effect was thought to be a possible explanation as to why there has been a dra-matic increase in allergy-related conditions such as asthma, eczema, and other hyperimmune response conditions in the omega-3-deficient modern era.

Dosages for Children

Although omega-3 EFA supplements for adults generally have more EPA than DHA, the opposite is true for children's supplements. Because the development of brain and eye tissue, in which DHA is the predominant EFA, is so rapid from about birth to age five, children in this age range should get at least 150 mg of DHA per day. With today's American diet loaded with mostly omega-6 EFAs, the typical child is getting only between 30 and 50 mg per day.

Formula-fed babies can get adequate amounts of DHA from supplemented formulas, and breast-fed babies will get the DHA they require from their moth-er's milk, provided the mother herself is getting adequate amounts of DHA. But once weaned, young children should be supplemented with dietary fish oil sup-plements if they are not consuming enough omega-3 EFAs in their diets. Gener-ally, the supplements for children contain both omega-3 and omega-6 EFAs in a balanced formulation, with approximately equal amounts of DHA and EPA.

Consuming fish-oil soft gel capsules can be difficult for children, and most manufacturers offer flavored fish oil for children.

POTENTIAL SIDE EFFECTS AND CONTRAINDICATIONS

We address here the most common side effects of supplementation with omega-3 EFA fish oils. Generally, there are very few if any ill effects, but of course if you experience any side effects, beyond the occasional loose stools, consult with your physician.

Allergies

People with a history of allergy or hypersensitivity to fish should avoid fish oil and any omega-3 EFA products derived from fish. In rare cases, skin rash, hives, and respiratory symptoms have been reported as side effects of fish oil supplementation.

Bleeding

Intake of 3 grams or more per day of omega-3 fatty acids may increase the risk of bleeding as per earlier reports in the literature, but this has been seen only in changes in the blood levels of the many factors that relate to clotting and has not been reported clinically in those with normal blood-clotting function. In other words, rarely has any excessive bleeding tendency been attributed to use of fish oil, but it needs to be considered as a potential problem, especially in higher dosing of 3 grams per day or more.

A 1998 study by S. L. Archer of more than 1,600 subjects who were evaluated for their EPA and DHA consumption found no change in the subjects' blood clotting factors no matter how much fish they consumed. Similarly, most studies investigating the relationship between fish consumption or fish oil supplementation and bleeding changes have also shown no significant increase in bleeding risk, but all have reported significant changes in blood values of clotting factors, which may result in some reduced clotting response. A study by E. B. Schmidt and colleagues in 1990 examined the dose-response effects of omega-3 EFAs on lipids and bleeding. Ten healthy males were each given 1.3 grams, 4 grams, or 9 grams of omega-3 polyunsaturated fatty acids daily for six-week periods. Their triglyceride levels were found to be reduced in a dose-dependent fashion. At 4 grams per day the subjects' bleeding time became slightly prolonged, and at 9 grams per day they had increased blood value changes, including bleeding time prolongation and plasminogen changes, but at no time did they experience spontaneous bleeding.

A study by M. Berrettini in 1996 evaluated forty subjects with chronic atherosclerotic disease (CAD) who were assigned 3 grams per day of EPA, DHA, or vegetable oil for sixteen weeks. Blood samples were drawn at three, eight, and sixteen weeks. The results of this study confirm the effectiveness of the omega-3 EFAs in reducing blood lipids, such as cholesterol and triglycerides. The CAD patients taking the omega-3 EFAs showed a decrease in the vascular clotting system, which may explain the anti-thrombotic (anti-clotting) activity of a fish-rich diet and fish oil derivatives.

Very large intakes of omega-3 fatty acids, in the range of 12 grams or more a day, may increase the risk of hemorrhagic (bleeding) stroke. As described in Chapter 5, in the 1970s Inuit Eskimos who consumed very large quantities of omega-3 EFAs were found to have a very low risk of heart disease and stroke from clotting but did report nosebleeds and blood in the urine. Blood work assessing clotting factors in these Eskimos showed a decrease in platelet aggregation, prolonged bleeding time, and increased fibrinolysis (breaking down of blood clots).

Generally, dosing of more than 3 grams of omega-3 EFAs is rarely needed. If such a high dosing is pursued for a medical condition, such as Crohn's disease or another autoimmune disease, it should be done under a physician's supervision.

Blood-Thinning Drugs and Omega-3 EFAs

The term *blood thinner* does not exist in medical terminology but is often used to describe drugs such as warfarin (Coumadin) and heparin, which are designed to reduce the body's ability to clot. These are complex drugs that are used in situations were the risk of clotting in a blood vessel, such as a coronary artery or a brain blood vessel, outweighs the serious risk of excessive bleeding and hemorrhage. These drugs must be monitored closely and the dose adjusted frequently to maintain the balance between too much clotting risk (thick blood) versus too much bleeding risk (thin blood). The measurement of this balance is called a prothrombin time (PT); often an INR (international normalized ratio), which allows blood values to be easily compared between labs, is also calculated and reported with the PT.

The fact is that this balance can be easily disturbed by many dietary factors, such as consumption of foods high in vitamin K. Fish oil supplements used in conjunction with warfarin can also disrupt this balance. Typically, most physicians do not allow patients on warfarin to take fish oil due to the fact it can increase the INR and result in potential bleeding complications. M. S. Buckley and colleagues reported in 2004 on a patient who doubled her fish oil dose from 1,000 to 2,000 mg per day. Without dietary, lifestyle, or medication changes, the INR increased from a relatively good level of 2.8 to a very high level of 4.3 within one month. The authors concluded that omega-3 EFAs may work by lowering thromboxane A_2 supplies within the platelets as well as decreasing clotting factor VII.

For these reasons we cannot recommend fish oil supplements to those on warfarin (Coumadin) or heparin. If you are taking a platelet inhibitor, such as aspirin or clopidogrel (Plavix), you can use fish oil safely, but such usage should be reviewed on a case-by-case basis with your doctor.

Gastrointestinal Upset

Gastrointestinal upset was a common complaint with many fish oils in the past. Because of the many changes in fish processing techniques and the increased concentrations of EPA and DHA, so that a lesser volume of fish oil is required, most of the gastrointestinal side effects have been significantly reduced. Diarrhea is rare and generally self-limiting, but if persistent, a reduction of the volume of oil usually will mitigate this side effect. Along with occasional burping, some people have complained of acid reflux, heartburn, and indigestion. Abdominal bloating and abdominal pain are rare; if they occur, it may indicate that the fish oil has turned rancid and should be discarded. Fishy aftertaste is common, but flavor additives can help, as can consuming fish oil with food.

Low Blood Pressure

As we reviewed in Chapter 5, many trials have reported small but significant reductions in blood pressure resulting from omega-3 EFA supplementation. Generally, these studies were done on hypertensive patients and helped to reduce the need for blood-pressure-lowering medication. The effects appear to be dose-responsive (higher doses have greater effects). In patients who already have low blood pressure, initial doses of fish oil should be small, with a gradual increase to watch for any symptoms of excessively low blood pressure (dizziness). This caution would also be appropriate for those taking blood-pressure-lowering medications.

Vitamin E, D, and A Levels

Many fish oil supplements have vitamin E added as an antioxidant to reduce spoilage and rancidity. If excessive amounts of additional vitamin E are consumed, or if the fish oil supplement has excessively high levels of vitamin E (the standard amount is generally 30 IU, or 100 percent of the daily requirement), elevated levels of this fat-soluble vitamin may result.

Cod liver oil contains both vitamins A and D, and therefore supplementation of these vitamins in conjunction with cod liver oil is not recommended, and the dosage guidelines given on the packaging of the oil should not be exceeded.

Glossary

Adhesion molecule. Any of a large number of cell-surface molecules of several different classes that affect the attachment of one cell to another.

Antibody. A protein produced by the immune system in response to an antigen, often a virus or *bacterium.*

Apolipoprotein. A protein that combines with a fat to form a *lipoprotein.* Apolipoprotein E (ApoE) forms the very-low-density lipoproteins (vLDL) used to remove excess cholesterol from the blood and carry it to the liver for processing. ApoE is also associated with several cardiovascular disorders.

Arrhythmia. Abnormal heart rhythm that relates to the electric control of the heartbeat. Arrhythmia can range in severity from minor to very serious; in some cases it can lead to sudden death.

Arteriosclerosis. The process by which the arteries change resulting in decreased elasticity, thickening of the blood vessel walls, and narrowing of the lumen (opening). It can eventually lead to complete blockage resulting in heart attack or stroke.

Arthritis. The inflammation of a joint.

Asthma. A chronic or acute condition causing difficulty in breathing. It is caused by overreaction of airways to irritants and constriction of small airways.

Atherosclerosis. One of many diseases in which fat builds up in the large- and medium-sized arteries, restricting blood flow. Similar to *arteriosclerosis.*

Autoimmune disease. A disorder in which the immune system mistakenly attacks and destroys body tissue that it believes to be foreign.

B cell. A cell found in bone marrow that becomes either a memory cell or a plasma cell that forms antibodies against a foreign substance.

Bacterium. A tiny, one-celled organism that reproduces by cell division and can be found in virtually any environment.

Basophil. A type of white blood cell that contains inflammatory mediators such as *histamine.*

Cancer. A disease caused by the abnormal and uncontrolled division of cells that invade and destroy surrounding body tissues.

Chemotaxis. Movement of a cell toward or away from a chemical substance.

Cholesterol. A fatty substance that higher organisms use in the construction of cell membranes and as an ingredient for making steroid molecules; it is carried through the bloodstream in molecules called *lipoproteins.*

Complement system. A set of molecules in the blood activated by the invasion of bacteria, injury, or other immune triggers, causing a response associated with starting and maintaining inflammation.

COX inhibitor. A drug that blocks the action of the *cyclooxygenase (COX)* enzyme.

C-reactive protein (CRP). A protein not normally found at high levels in the blood of healthy people; when present, it indicates inflammation in the body.

Cyclooxygenase (COX). An enzyme used to convert fatty acids found in cell membranes into eicosanoids. It is also the enzyme that is the molecular target of *nonsteroidal anti-inflammatory drugs (NSAIDs).*

Cytokine. A molecule that controls reactions among cells; key component of inflammation.

Dermis. The skin layer just beneath the *epidermis;* it is composed of connective tissue and blood vessels.

Edema. Swelling caused by the excessive accumulation of fluid in body tissues.

Eicosanoid. A class of molecules converted from the fatty acids found in cell membranes. Like hormones, they function as chemical messengers in the body. They stimulate both inflammatory and anti-inflammatory mechanisms, along with several other actions.

Endogenous. Arising within the body or derived from the body.

Endothelium. A layer of cells lining the inside of blood vessels and the heart.

Eosinophil. Amoeba-like scavenger white blood cell that consumes cellular debris and is often involved in allergic responses.

Epidermis. Outer layer of skin.

Epithelial cell. See *epithelium.*

Epithelium. A layer of cells that covers the internal and external surfaces of the body, including cavities, ducts, and vessels.

Exogenous. From outside the body.

Free radical. An unstable molecule that reacts quickly with other atoms and molecules and can cause damage to living tissues. The oxygen free radical is the most common one.

Gene expression. The translation of information encoded in a gene and expressed or made into protein or RNA.

Histamine. A molecule released especially during an allergic response that causes smooth muscle contraction, inflammation, mucus secretion, and other allergy symptoms.

Immune system. The body's system for protection against infection and disease; involves immune cells, antibodies, and other molecules.

Infection (bacterial, viral). Invasion of the body by harmful microorganisms such as viruses, bacteria, fungi, or parasites.

Inflammation. The body's immediate, defensive reaction to any injury.

Inflammation mediator. Molecule inside or outside the body that plays a role in inflammation.

Insulin. A hormone produced in the pancreas that helps control levels of sugars, fats, and proteins in the body.

Interferon. A molecule produced by a cell infected with a virus that helps the body fight off viral infections.

Interleukin. One of a class of *inflammation mediators.*

Ischemia. Lack of oxygen to a cell, either acute or chronic, which can result in cell death or injury. Associated with blood vessel blockage, as in the case of a heart attack or stroke.

Leukocytes. White blood cells that exist as several types in the body and that act as a part of the immune system by destroying invading cells and removing cellular debris, among some of their many functions.

Leukotriene. An inflammatory eicosanoid that is known to be responsible, among other effects, for allergic responses that can cause lung constriction and muscle contraction.

Lipoprotein. A molecule made of a protein connected to a fat. Lipoproteins transport cholesterol and other fats through the bloodstream.

Lymphocyte. A type of white blood cell found in lymphatic tissue that is used for immune responses to produce antibodies (B cells and T cells).

Macrophage. A type of white blood cell that can consume bacteria (in a process called phagocytosis) and cellular debris during inflammation and can produce inflammatory molecules.

Mast cell. A type of white blood cell found in tissues that produces *histamine* and other inflammatory molecules.

Monocyte. A type of white blood cell that can consume bacteria (in a process called phagocytosis) and that breaks down debris and invading cells. A mature monocyte is a *macrophage* cell.

Multiple sclerosis. Autoimmune disease in which the body attacks its own nervous system, destroying the myelin sheath that protects nerve cells.

Myelin. A protein that covers and acts as an electrical insulator for nerve fibers.

Nerve disorder. Any of a variety of health disorders affecting the brain, spinal cord, and nervous system.

Neuron. A nerve cell consisting of a cell body, an axon, axon terminals, and dendrites; it receives and conducts electrical impulses from the brain.

Neutrophil. A type of white blood cell that travels through the blood to an injured site, generally in response to the signaling of chemical messengers released by the injured tissue (*chemotaxis*), and that can destroy invading bacteria.

Nitric oxide. A highly reactive gas that is involved in a wide array of biological functions, such as blood vessel dilation, and that functions as a part of the body's immune system.

Nonsteroidal anti-inflammatory drug (NSAID). Any of a class of drugs that reduces pain, fever, or inflammation by interfering with the synthesis of inflammatory eicosanoids (prostaglandins).

Pathogen. Microorganism that causes disease.

Plasma. Blood serum, in which the blood cells float, that also contains clotting factors.

Platelet. A piece of tissue made from a larger blood cell that is found in the bloodstream and is responsible, along with other factors, for the blood-clotting process.

Prostaglandin. A type of eicosanoid that can, among many diverse functions, stimulate inflammation.

Protein. A large molecule used for the structure, function, and regulation of the body's cells, tissues, and organs.

Serum. The liquid component of blood.

Stenosis. Any type of narrowing; generally associated with a blood vessel or canal, such as the spinal canal.

Systemic inflammation. Inflammation throughout the body.

T cell. A type of cell produced by the thymus and active in immune reactions.

Thrombosis. The formation of a clot (thrombus) inside a blood vessel, blocking the flow of blood through that vessel.

Thromboxane. A type of *eicosanoid* that can, among many diverse functions, stimulate vasoconstriction and the clumping of platelets, resulting in a clot.

Tumor necrosis factor (TNF). A *cytokine* produced primarily by monocytes and macrophages that is associated with acute inflammatory response.

Triglyceride. A type of fat, found in vegetable oils and animal fats, that is composed of one glycerol molecule and three fatty acids. This shape is most stable and allows for the transport of fatty acids in the blood.

Virus. Infectious agent composed of a protein coat around a DNA or RNA core; to reproduce, viruses depend on living cells.

References

Abdi-Dezfuli F, Froyland L, Thorsen T, Aakvaag A, Berge RK. Eicosanpentaenoic acid and sulphur substituted fatty acid analogues inhibit the proliferation of human breast cancer cells in culture. *Breast Cancer Res Treat.* 1997;45:229–239.

Abou-El-Ela SH, Prasse KW, Farrell RL, Carroll RW, Wade AE, Bunce OR. Effects of D,L-2-difuoromethylornithine and indomethacin on mammary tumor promotion in rats fed high n-3 and/or n-6 fat diets. *Cancer Res.* 1989;49:1434–1440.

Adam O. Dietary fatty acids and immune reactions in synovial tissue. *Eur J Med Res.* 2003;8(8):381–387.

Agranoff BW, Goldberg D. Diet and the geographical distribution of multiple sclerosis. *Lancet.* 1974;2(7888):1061–1066.

Albert CM, Campos H, Stampfer MJ, et al. Blood levels of long-chain n-3 fatty acids and the risk of sudden death. *N Engl J Med.* 2002;346:1113–1118.

Albert CM, Hennekens CH, O'Donnell CJ, et al. Fish consumption and risk of sudden cardiac death. *JAMA.* 1998;279:23–28.

Alexander JW, Levy A, Custer D, et al. Arginine, fish oil, and donor-specific transfusions independently improve cardiac allograft survival in rats given subtherapeutic doses of cyclosporin. *JPEN J Parenter Enteral Nutr.* May 1998;22(3):152–155.

Aman MG, Mitchell EA, Turbott SH. The effects of essential fatty-acid supplementation by Efamol in hyperactive-children. *J Abnorm Child Psychol.* 1987;15:75–90.

Anderson TJ, Meredith IT, Yeung AC, Frei B, Selwyn AP, Ganz P. The effect of cholesterol-lowering and antioxidant therapy on endothelium-dependent coronary vasomotion. *N Engl J Med.* 1995;332:488–493.

Andreassen AK, Hartmann A, Offstad J, et al. Hypertension prophylaxis with omega-3 fatty acids in heart transplant recipients. *J Am Coll Cardiol.* 1997;29(6):1324–1331.

Anti M, Marra G, Armelao F, et al. Effect of omega-3 fatty acids on rectal mucosal cell proliferation in subjects at risk for colon cancer. *Gastroenterology.* September 1992; 103:883–891.

Appel LJ, Miller ER III, Seidler AJ, Whelton PK. Does supplementation of diet with "fish oil" reduce blood pressure? A meta-analysis of controlled clinical trials. *Arch Intern Med.* 1993;153:1429–1438.

Archer SL, Green D, Chamberlain M, Dyer AR, Liu K. Association of dietary fish and n-3 fatty acid intake with hemostatic factors in the Coronary Artery Risk Development in Young Adults (CARDIA) Study. *Arterioscler Thromb Vasc Biol.* 1998;18:1119–1123.

Arm JP, Horton CE, Mencia-Huerta JM, et al. Effect of dietary supplementation with fish oil lipids on mild asthma. *Thorax.* 1988;43(2):84–92.

Arm JP, Horton CE, Spur BW, et al. The effects of dietary supplementation with fish oil lipids on the airways response to inhaled allergen in bronchial asthma. *Am Rev Respir Dis.* 1989;139(6):1395–1400.

Armstrong B, Doll R. Environmental factors and cancer incidence and mortality in different countries, with special reference to dietary practices. *Int J Cancer.* 1975;15: 617–631.

Ascherio A, Rimm EB, Giovannucci EL, Spiegelman D, Stampfer M, Willett WC. Dietary fat and risk of coronary heart disease in men: Cohort follow-up study in the United States. *BMJ.* 1996;313(7049):84–90.

Ashley JM, Lowe NJ, Borok ME, Alfin-Slater RB. Fish oil supplementation results in decreased hypertriglyceridemia in patients with psoriasis undergoing etretinate or acitretin therapy. *J Am Acad Dermatol.* 1988;19:76–82.

Aslan A, Triadafilopoulos G. Fish oil fatty acid supplementation in active ulcerative colitis: A double-blind, placebo-controlled, crossover study. *Am J Gastroenterol.* 1992; 87(4):432–437.

Aucamp AK, Schoeman HS, Coetzee JH. Pilot trial to determine the efficacy of a low dose of fish oil in the treatment of angina pectoris in the geriatric patient. *Prostaglandins Leukot Essent Fatty Acids.* 1993;49(3):687–689.

Augustsson K, Michaud DS, Rimm EB, et al. A prospective study of intake of fish and marine fatty acids and prostate cancer. *Cancer Epidemiol Biomarkers Prev.* 2003;12(1): 64–67.

Axerold L. Omega-3 fatty acids in diabetes mellitus: Gift from the sea. *Diabetes.* 1989;38:539–543.

Badalamenti S, Salerno F, Lorenzano E, et al. Renal effects of dietary supplementation with fish oil in cyclosporine-treated liver transplant recipients. *Hepatology.* December 1995;22(6):1695–1671.

Bagga D, Capone S, Wang H-J, Heber D, Lill M, Chap L, Glaspy JA. Dietary modulation of omega-3/omega-6 polyunsaturated fatty acid rations in patients with breast cancer. *J Natl Cancer Inst.* 1997;89:1123–1131.

Bagga D, Wang L, Farias-Eisner R, Glaspy JA, Reddy ST. Differential effects of prostaglandin derived from ω-6 and ω-3 polyunsaturated fatty acids on COX-2 expression and IL-6 secretion. *Proc Nat Acad Sci USA.* 2003;100:1751–1756.

Bakker DJ, Haberstroh BN, Philbrick DJ, et al. Triglyceride lowering in nephrotic syndrome patients consuming a fish oil concentrate. *Nutrit Res.* 1989;9:27–34.

Bakker N, van't Veer P, Zock PL, et al. Adipose fatty acids and cancers of the breast, prostate and colon: An ecological study. *Int J Cancer.* 1997;72:587–591.

Balestrieri GP, Maffi V, Sleiman I, et al. Fish oil supplementation in patients with heterozygous familial hypercholesterolemia. *Recenti Prog Med.* 1996;87(3):102–105.

Bang H, Dyerberg J, Hjorne N. The composition of food consumed by Greenland Eskimos. *Acta Med Scand.* 1976;200:69–73.

Barber MD, McMillan DC, Preston T, et al. Metabolic response to feeding in weight-losing pancreatic cancer patients and its modulation by a fish-oil-enriched nutritional supplement. *Clin Sci* (Lond). 2000;98:389–399.

Barber MD, Ross JA, Preston T, et al. Fish oil-enriched nutritional supplement attenuates progression of the acute-phase response in weight-losing patients with advanced pancreatic cancer. *J Nutr.* 1999;129(6):1120–1125.

Barber MD, Ross JA, Voss AC, et al. The effect of an oral nutritional supplement enriched with fish oil on weight-loss in patients with pancreatic cancer. *Br J Cancer.* 1999;81(1):80–86.

Barberger-Gateau P, Letenneur L, Deschamps V, et al. Fish, meat, and risk of dementia: Cohort study. *BMJ.* 2002;325(7370):932–933.

Beckermann B, Beneke M, Seitz I. Comparative bioavailability of eicosapentaenoic acid and docasahexaenoic acid from triglycerides, free fatty acids and ethyl esters in volunteers. *Arzneimittelforschung.* June 1990;40(6):700–704.

Beckles WI, Elliott TM, Everard ML. Omega-3 fatty acids (from fish oils) for cystic fibrosis. *Cochrane Database Syst Rev.* 2002;(3):CD002201.

Belayev L, Marcheselli VL, Khoutorova L, et al. Docosahexaenoic acid complexed to albumin elicits high-grade ischemic neuroprotection. *Stroke.* 2005;36:118.

Belluzzi A, Brignola C, Boschi S, et al. A novel enteric coated preparation of omega-3 fatty acids in a group of steroid-dependent ulcerative colitis: An open study [abstract]. *Gastroenterology.* 1997;112(suppl):A930.

Belluzzi A, Brignola C, Campieri M, et al. Effects of new fish oil derivative on fatty acid phospholipid-membrane pattern in a group of Crohn's disease patients. *Dig Dis Sci.* 1994;39(12):2589–2594.

Belluzzi A, Brignola C, Campieri M, Pera A, Boschi S, Miglioli M. Effect of an enteric-coated fish-oil preparation on relapses in Crohn's disease. *N Engl J Med.* 1996;334: 1557–1560.

Bemelmans WJ, Broer J, Feskens EJ, et al. Effect of an increased intake of alpha-linolenic acid and group nutritional education on cardiovascular risk factors: The Mediterranean Alpha-linolenic Enriched Groningen Dietary Intervention (MARGARIN) Study. *Am J Clin Nutr.* 2002;75(2):221–227.

Bennett WM, Carpenter CB, Shapiro ME, et al. Delayed omega-3 fatty acid supplements in renal transplantation: A double-blind, placebo-controlled study. *Transplantation.* 1995;59(3):352–356.

Berrettini M, Parise P, Ricotta S, Iorio A, Peirone C, Nenci GG. Increased plasma levels of tissue factor pathway inhibitor (TFPI) after n-3 polyunsaturated fatty acids supplementation in patients with chronic atherosclerotic disease. *Thromb Haemost.* March 1996;75(3):395–400.

Berthoux FC, Guerin C, Burgard G, et al. One-year randomized controlled trial with omega-3 fatty acid-fish oil in clinical renal transplantation. *Transplant Proc.* 1992;24(6): 2578-2582.

Best, Ben. (1990) "Fats You Need—Essential Fatty Acids." Retrieved December, 2006. www.benbest.com/health/essfat.html.

Bilo HJK, Homan van der Heide JJ, Gans RO, Donker HJ. Omega-3 polyunsaturated fatty acids in chronic renal insufficiency. *Nephron.* 1991;57(4):385-393.

Birch DG, Birch EE, Hoffman DR, et al. Retinal development in very-low-birth-weight infants fed diets differing in omega-3 fatty acids. *Invest Ophthalmol Vis Sci.* 1992; 33(8): 2365-2376.

Birch EE, Birch DG, Hoffman DR, et al. Dietary essential fatty acid supply and visual acuity development. *Invest Ophthalmol Vis Sci.* 1992;33(11):3242-3253.

Biscione F, Totteri A, De Vita A, Lo Bianco F, Altamura G. Effect of omega-3 fatty acids on the prevention of atrial arrhythmias. *Ital Heart J Suppl.* 2005;6(1):53-59.

Bittiner SB, Tucker WF, Bleehen S. Fish oil in psoriasis: A double-blind randomized placebo-controlled trial. *Br J Dermatol.* 1987;117:25-26.

Bittiner SB, Tucker WF, Cartwright I, et al. A double-blind, randomised, placebo-controlled trial of fish oil in psoriasis. *Lancet.* 1988;1:378-380.

Bjerregaard P, Mulvad G, Pedersen HS. Cardiovascular risk factors in Inuit of Greenland. *Int J Epidemiol.* 1997;26:1182-1190.

Bjerve K, Brubaak AM, Fougner K, Johnsen H, Midthjell K, Vik T. Omega-3 fatty acids: Essential fatty acids with important biological effects, and serum phospholipid fatty acids as markers of dietary 3-fatty acid intake. *Am J Clin Nutr.* 1993;57(suppl):801S-6S.

Bjorneboe A, Smith AK, Bjorneboe GE, et al. Effect of dietary supplementation with n-3 fatty acids on clinical manifestations of psoriasis. *Br J Dermatol.* 1988;118(1):77-83.

Bjorneboe A, Soyland E, Bjorneboe GE, et al. Effect of dietary supplementation with eicosapentaenoic acid in the treatment of atopic dermatitis. *Br J Dermatol.* 1987;117(4): 463-469.

Bjorneboe A, Soyland E, Bjorneboe GE, et al. Effect of n-3 fatty acid supplement to patients with atopic dermatitis. *J Intern Med Suppl.* 1989;225(731):233-236.

Blanchet C, Dewailly E, Ayotte P, Bruneau S, Receveur O, Holub BJ. Contribution of selected traditional and market foods to the diet of Nunavik Inuit women. *Can J Diet Pract Res.* 2000;61:50-59.

Bonaa KH, Bjerve KS, Straume B, et al. Effect of eicosapentaenoic and docosahexaenoic acids on blood pressure in hypertension: A population-based intervention trial from the Tromso Study. *N Engl J Med.* 1990;322(12):795-801.

Bordin L, Prianti G, Musacchio E, et al. Arachidonic acid-induced IL-6 expression is mediated by PKC-alpha activation in osteoblastic cells. *Biochem.* 2003;42:4485-4491.

Bougnoux P, Koscielny S, Chajes V, Descamps P, Couet C, Calais G. Alpha-linolenic acid content of adipose breast tissue: A host determinant of the risk of early metastasis in breast cancer. *Br J Canc.* 1993;70:330-334.

Bower JH, Maraganore DM, McDonnell SK, Rocca WA. Incidence and distribution of parkinsonism in Olmsted County, Minnesota, 1976-1990. *Neurology.* 1999;52:1214-1220.

Boyd NF, Connelly P, Lynch H, et al. Plasma lipids, lipoproteins, and familial breast cancer. *Cancer Epidemiol Biomarkers Prev.* 1995;4:117–122.

Boyd NF, Greenberg C, Lockwood G, et al. Effects at two years of a low-fat, high-carbohydrate diet on radiologic features of the breast: Results from a randomized trial. *J Natl Cancer Inst.* 1997;89:488–498.

Boyd NF, Lockwood GA, Byng JW, Tritchler DL, Yaffe MJ. Mammographic densities and breast cancer risk. *Cancer Epidemiol Biomarkers Prev.* 1998;7:1133–1144.

Boyd NF, Martin LJ, Noffel M, Lockwood GA, Tritchler DL. A meta-analysis of studies of dietary fat and breast cancer risk. *Br J Cancer.* 1993;68:627–636.

Boyd NF, Martin L, Lockwood G, Greenberg C, Yaffe M, Tritchler D. Diet and breast cancer. *Nutr Epidemiol.* 1998;14:722–724.

Braden LM, Carroll KK. Dietary polyunsaturated fat in relation to mammary carcinogenesis in rats. *Lipids.* 1986;21:285–288.

Brassard P, Robinson E, Lavallée C. Prevalence of diabetes mellitus among the James Bay Cree of northern Quebec. *Can Med Assoc J.* 1993;149:303–307.

Bresalier RS, Sandler RS, Quan H, et al. The Adenomatous Polyp Prevention on Vioxx (APPROVe): Cardiovascular events associated with rofecoxib in a colorectal adenoma chemoprevention trial. *N Engl J Med.* 2005;352:1092–1102.

Brouwer RM, Wenting GJ, Pos B, et al. Fish oil ameliorates established cyclosporin A nephrotoxicity after heart transplantation [abstract]. *Kidney Int.* 1991;40:347–348.

Bruera E, Strasser F, Palmer JL, et al. Effect of fish oil on appetite and other symptoms in patients with advanced cancer and anorexia/cachexia: A double-blind, placebo-controlled study. *J Clin Oncol.* 2003;21(1):129–134.

Bucher HC, Hengstler P, Schindler C, et al. N-3 polyunsaturated fatty acids in coronary heart disease: A meta-analysis of randomized controlled trials. *Am J Med.* 2002; 112(4): 298–304.

Buckley MS, Goff AD, Knapp WE. Fish oil interaction with warfarin. *Ann Pharmacother.* 2004;38(1):50–52.

Bulliyya G, Reddy KK, Reddy GP, Reddanna P, KumariI KS. Lipid profiles among fish-consuming coastal and non-fish-consuming inland populations. *Eur J Clin Nutr.* 1990; 44:481–485.

Bulstra-Ramakers MT, Huisjes HJ, Visser GH. The effects of 3g eicosapentaenoic acid daily on recurrence of intrauterine growth retardation and pregnancy induced hypertension. *BJOG.* 1994;102:123–126.

Burdge GC, Wootton SA. Conversion of alpha-linolenic acid to eicosapentaenoic, docosapentaenoic and docosahexaenoic acids in young women. *Br J Nutr.* 2002;88:411–420.

Burgess JR, Stevens L, Zhang W, Peck L. Long-chain polyunsaturated fatty acids in children with attention-deficit hyperactivity disorder. *Am J Clin Nutr.* 2000;71(1; suppl): 327S–330S.

Burr GO, Burr MM. On the nature and role of the fatty acids essential in nutrition. *J Biol Chem.* 1930;86(Jan. 9):587.

Burr ML, Ashfield-Watt PA, Dunstan FD, et al. Lack of benefit of dietary advice to men with angina: Results of a controlled trial. *Eur J Clin Nutr.* 2003;57:193–200.

Burr ML, Fehily AM, Gilbert JF, et al. Effects of changes in fat, fish, and fibre intakes on death and myocardial reinfarction: Diet and Reinfarction Trial (DART). *Lancet.* 1989; 2:757–761.

Burr ML, Sweetham PM, Fehily AM. Diet and reinfarction. *Eur Heart J.* 1994;15(8): 1152–1153.

Byers T, Rock CL, Hamilton KK. Dietary changes after breast cancer: What should we recommend? *Cancer Pract.* 1997;5:317–320.

Cade J, Thomas E, Vail A. Case-control study of breast cancer in south east England: Nutritional factors. *J Epidemiol Community Health.* 1998;52:105–110.

Cairns JA, Gill J, Morton B, et al. Fish oils and low-molecular-weight heparin for the reduction of restenosis after percutaneous transluminal coronary angioplasty: The EMPAR Study. *Circulation.* 1996;94(7):1553–1560.

Calabrese JR, Rapport DJ, Shelton MD. Fish oils and bipolar disorder: A promising but untested treatment. *Arch Gen Psychiatry.* 1999;56(5):413–414.

Calder PC. Dietary fatty acids and the immune system. *Nutr Rev.* 1998;56:S70–S83.

Calder PC. N-3 polyunsaturated fatty acids and inflammation: From molecular biology to the clinic. *Lipids.* 2003;38:342–352.

Caleffi M, Ashraf J, Rowe PH, Thomas BS, Fentiman IS. A comparison of the fatty acid profiles of subcutaneous fat from women with breast cancer, benign breast disease and normal controls. *Anticancer Res.* 1987;7:1305–1308.

Calo L, Bianconi L, Colivicchi F, et al. N-3 fatty acids for the prevention of atrial fibrillation after coronary artery bypass surgery: A randomized, controlled trial. *J Am Coll Cardiol.* 2005;45(10):1723–1728.

Calon F, Lim GP, Yang F, et al. Docosahexaenoic acid protects from dendritic pathology in an Alzheimer's disease mouse model. *Neuron.* 2004;43(5):633–645.

Camandola S, Leonarduzzi G, Musso T, et al. Nuclear factor κB is activated by arachidonic acid but not by eicosapentenoic acid. *Biochem Biophys Res Commun.* 1996; 229:643–647.

Capone ML, Tacconelli S, Sciulli MG, et al. Clinical pharmacology of platelet, monocyte, and vascular cyclooxygenase inhibition by naproxen and low-dose aspirin in healthy subjects. *Circulation.* 2004;109:1468–1471.

Capone SL, Bagga D, Glaspy JA. Relationship between omega-3 and omega-6 fatty acid ratios and breast cancer. *Nutrition.* 1997;13:822–823.

Carlson SE, Werkman SH. A randomized trial of visual attention of preterm infants fed docosahexaenoic acid until two months. *Lipids.* 1996;31(1):85–90.

Carlson SE, Werkman SH, Rhodes PG, et al. Visual-acuity development in healthy preterm infants: Effect of marine-oil supplementation. *Am J Clin Nutr.* 1993;58(1):35–42.

Carlson SE, Werkman SH, Tolley EA. Effect of long-chain n-3 fatty acid supplementation on visual acuity and growth of preterm infants with and without bronchopulmonary dysplasia. *Am J Clin Nutr.* 1996;63(5):687–697.

Carragee EJ. Persistent low back pain. *N Engl J Med.* 2005;352:1891–1898.

Carroll KK. The role of dietary fat in breast cancer. *Curr Opin Lipidol.* 1997;8:53–56.

Carroll KK, Khor HT. Effects of level and type of dietary fat on incidence of mammary tumors induced by 7,12-dimethylbenz(a)anthracene. *Lipids.* 1971;6:415–420.

Castelli WP. The triglyceride issue: A view from Framingham. *Am Heart J.* 1986;112: 432–437.

Castelli WP, Wilson PW, Levy D, Anderson K. Cardiovascular risk factors in the elderly. *Am J Cardiol.* 1989;63(suppl):12H–19H.

Cave WT. Dietary omega-3 polyunsaturated fats and breast cancer. *Nutrition.* 1996;12(suppl):S39–S56.

Cave WT. Omega-3 polyunsaturated fatty acids in rodent models of breast cancer. *Breast Cancer Res Treat.* 1997;46:239–246.

Caygill CPJ, Charlett A, Hill MJ. Fat, fish, fish oil and cancer. *Br J Cancer.* 1996; 74:159–164.

Caygill CPJ, Hill MJ. Fish, n-3 fatty acids and human colorectal and breast cancer mortality. *Eur J Cancer Prev.* 1995;4:329–332.

Chajes V, Niyongabo T, Lanson M, Fignon A, Couet C, Bougnoux P. Fatty-acid composition of breast and iliac adipose tissue in breast cancer patients. *Int J Cancer.* 1991; 50:405–408.

Chajes V, Sattler W, Stranzl A, Kostner GM. Influence of n-3 fatty acids on the growth of human breast cancer cells in vitro: Relationship to peroxides and vitamin-E. *Breast Cancer Res Treat.* 1995;34:199–212.

Chan DC, Watts GF, Barrett PH, et al. Effect of atorvastatin and fish oil on plasma high-sensitivity C-reactive protein concentrations in individuals with visceral obesity. *Clin Chem.* 2002;48(6; part 1):877–883.

Cheuvront SN. The Zone Diet phenomenon: A closer look at the science behind the claims. *J Am Coll Nutr.* 2003;22(1):9–17.

Chiu CC, Huang SY, Shen WW, et al. Omega-3 fatty acids for depression in pregnancy. *Am J Psychiatry.* 2003;160(2):385.

Christensen JH, Gustenhoff P, Ejlersen E, et al. N-3 fatty acids and ventricular extrasystoles in patients with ventricular tachyarrhythmias. *Nutr Res.* 1995;15(1):1-8.

Christensen JH, Gustenhoff P, Korup E, et al. Effect of fish oil on heart rate variability in survivors of myocardial infarction: A double blind randomised controlled trial. *BMJ.* 1996;312(7032):677–678.

Clark WF, Parbtani A. Omega-3 fatty acid supplementation in clinical and experimental lupus nephritis. *Am J Kidney Dis.* 1994;23(5):644–647.

Clark WF, Parbtani A, Naylor CD, et al. Fish oil in lupus nephritis: Clinical findings and methodological implications. *Kidney Int.* 1993;44(1):75–86.

Clarke JT, Cullen-Dean G, Regelink E, et al. Increased incidence of epistaxis in adolescents with familial hypercholesterolemia treated with fish oil. *J Pediatr.* 1990;116(1): 139–141.

Clarke SD. Polyunsaturated fatty acid regulation of gene transcription: A mechanism to improve energy balance and insulin resistance. *Br J Nutr.* 2000;83(suppl):S59–S66.

Clarke SD, Jump DB. Dietary polyunsaturated fatty acid regulation of gene transcription. *Annu Rev Nutr.* 1994;14:83–98.

Cleland LG, French JK, Betts WH, Murphy GA, Elliott MJ. Clinical and biochemical effects of dietary fish oil supplements in rheumatoid arthritis. *J Rheumatol.* 1988;15: 1471–1475.

Cobiac L, Nestel PJ, Wing LM, et al. A low-sodium diet supplemented with fish oil lowers blood pressure in the elderly. *J Hypertens.* 1992;10(1):87–92.

Cohen LA, Chen-Backlund J-Y, Sepkovic DW, Sugie S. Effect of varying proportions of dietary menhaden and corn oil on experimental rat mammary tumor promotion. *Lipids.* 1993;28:449–456.

Colditz GA. Fat, estrogens, and the time frame for prevention of breast cancer. *Epidemiology.* 1995;6:209–211.

Connor WE. Importance of n-3 fatty acids in health and disease. *Am J Clin Nutr.* 2000;71(1; suppl):171S–175S.

Connor WE. N-3 fatty acids from fish and fish oil: Panacea or nostrum? *Am J Clin Nutr.* October 2001;74(4):415–416.

Connor WE, Prince MJ, Ullmann D, et al. The hypotriglyceridemic effect of fish oil in adult-onset diabetes without adverse glucose control. *Ann N Y Acad Sci.* 1993;683: 337–340.

Conquer J, Cheryk L, Chan E, Gentry P, Holub B. Effect of supplementation with dietary seal oil on selected cardiovascular risk factors and hemostatic variables in healthy male subjects. *Thromb Res.* 1999;96:239–250.

Contacos C, Barter PJ, Sullivan DR. Effect of pravastatin and omega-3 fatty acids on plasma lipids and lipoproteins in patients with combined hyperlipidemia. *Arterioscler Thromb.* 1993;13:1755–1762.

Cotter J, Wooltorton E. New restrictions on celecoxib (Celebrex) use and the withdrawal of valdecoxib (Bextra). *Can Med Assoc J.* 2005;172:1299.

Cox ER, Frisse M, Behm A, Fairman KA. Over-the-counter pain reliever and aspirin use within a sample of long-term cyclooxygenase 2 users. *Arch Intern Med.* 2004;164: 1243–1246.

Craig-Schmidt M, White MT, Teer P, Johnson J, Lane HW. Menhaden, coconut, and corn oils and mammary tumor incidence in BALB/c virgin female mice treated with DMBA. *Nutr Cancer.* 1993;20:99–106.

Curtis CL, Harwood JL, Dent CM, Caterson B. Biological basis for the benefit of nutraceutical supplementation in arthritis. *Drug Discov Today.* 2004;9(4):165–172.

Curtis CL, Hughes CD, Flannery CR, Little CB, Harwood JL, Caterson B. N-3 fatty acids specifically modulate catabolic factors involved in articular cartilage degradation. *J Biol Chem.* 2000;275(2):721–724.

Curtis CL, Rees SG, Little CB, et al. Pathologic indicators of degradation and inflammation in human osteoarthritic cartilage are abrogated by exposure to n-3 fatty acids. *Arth Rheum.* 2002;46:1544–1553.

D'Almeida A, Carter JP, Anatol A, et al. Effects of a combination of evening primrose oil (gamma linolenic acid) and fish oil (eicosapentaenoic + docahexaenoic acid) versus magnesium, and versus placebo in preventing pre-eclampsia. *Women Health.* 1992; 19(2–3):117–131.

Dandona P, Aljada A, Chaudhuri A, Bandyopadhyay A. The potential influence of inflammation and insulin resistance on the pathogenesis and treatment of atherosclerosis-related complications in type 2 diabetes. *J Clin Endocrinol Metab.* 2003;88(6): 2422–2429.

Danno K, Sugie N. Combination therapy with low-dose etretinate and eicosapentaenoic acid for psoriasis vulgaris. *J Dermatol.* 1998;25(11):703–705.

Das UN. Essential fatty acid metabolism in patients with essential hypertension, diabetes mellitus and coronary heart disease. *Prostaglandins Leukot Essent Fatty Acids.* June 1995;52(6):387–91.

Das UN. Tumoricidal action of cis-unsaturated fatty acids and their relationship to free radicals and lipid peroxidation. *Cancer Lett.* 1991;56:235–243.

Das UN, Madhavi N, Sravan Kumar G, Padma M, Sangeetha P. Can tumour cell drug resistance be reversed by essential fatty acids and their metabolites? *Prostaglandins Leukot Essent Fatty Acids.* January 1998;58(1):39–54.

Daviglus ML, Stamler J, Orencia AJ, et al. Fish consumption and the 30-year risk of fatal myocardial infarction. *N Engl J Med.* 1997;336(15):1046–1053.

de Deckere EA. Possible beneficial effect of fish and fish n-3 polyunsaturated fatty acids in breast and colorectal cancer. *Eur J Cancer Prev.* 1999;8(3):213–221.

de Lau LML, Bornebroek M, Witteman JCM, Hofman A, Koudstaal PJ, Breteler MMB. Dietary fatty acids and the risk of Parkinson disease: The Rotterdam Study. *Neurology.* 2005;64:2040–2045

de Lorgeril M, Salen P, Martin JL, et al. Mediterranean diet, traditional risk factors, and the rate of cardiovascular complications after myocardial infarction: Final report of the Lyon Diet Heart Study. *Circulation.* 1999;99(6):779–785.

Demark-Wahnefried W, Rimer BK, Winer EP. Weight gain in women diagnosed with breast cancer. *J Am Diet Assoc.* 1997;97:519–526,529.

de Rijk MC, Breteler MM, Graveland GA, et al. Prevalence of Parkinson's disease in the elderly: The Rotterdam Study. *Neurology.* 1995;45:2143–2146.

de Roos NM, Bots ML, Katan MB. Replacement of dietary saturated fatty acids by trans fatty acids lowers serum HDL cholesterol and impairs endothelial function in healthy men and women. *Arterioscler Thromb Vasc Biol.* July 2001;21(7):1233–1237.

Després JP. Abdominal obesity and the risk of coronary artery disease. *Can J Cardiol.* 1992;8:561–562.

Després JP, Lamarche B, Mauriège P, et al. Hyperinsulinemia as an independent risk factor for ischemic heart disease. *N Engl J Med.* 1996;334:952–957.

Després JP, Morjani S, Lupien PJ, Tremblay A, Nadeau A, Bouchard C. Regional distribution of body fat, plasma lipoproteins, and cardiovascular disease. *Arteriosclerosis.* 1990; 10:497–511.

de Stefani E, Deneo-Pellegrini H, Mendilaharsu M, Ronco A. Essential fatty acids and breast cancer: A case-control study in Uruguay. *Int J Cancer.* 1997;76:491–494.

Deutch B. Menstrual pain in Danish women correlated with low n-3 polyunsaturated fatty acid intake. *Eur J Clin Nutr.* 1995;49:508–516.

Deutch B. [Painful menstruation and low intake of n-3 fatty acids]. *Ugeskr Laeger.* 1996; 158(29):4195–4198. [Article in Danish.]

Deutch B, Jorgensen EB, Hansen JC. Menstrual discomfort in Danish women reduced by dietary supplements of omega-3 PUFA and B12 (fish oil or seal oil capsules). *Nutr Res.* 2000;20(5):621–631.

De Vizia B, Raia V, Spano C, et al. Effect of an 8-month treatment with omega-3 fatty acids (eicosapentaenoic and docosahexaenoic) in patients with cystic fibrosis. *JPEN J Parenter Enteral Nutr.* 2003;27(1):52–57.

Dewailly E, Ayotte P, Blanchet C, et al. Weighing contaminant risks and nutrient benefits of country food in Nunavik. *Arctic Med Res.* 1996;55:13–19.

Dewailly E, Blanchet C, Gingras S, et al. Relations between n-3 fatty acid status and cardiovascular disease risk factors among Quebecers. *Am J Clin Nutr.* 2001;74(5):603–611.

Dewailly E, Blanchet C, Lemieux S, et al. N-3 fatty acids and cardiovascular disease risk factors among the Inuit of Nunavik. *Am J Clin Nutr.* 2001;74(4):464–473.

Dewailly E, Bruneau S, Laliberté C, et al. The contaminants. In: *Report of the Santé Québec Health Survey among the Inuit of Nunavik* (1992). Montreal: Ministère de la Santé et des Services Sociaux, Gouvernement du Québec; 1994:73–107.

Dewsbury CE, Graham P, Darley CR. Topical eicosapentaenoic acid (EPA) in the treatment of psoriasis. *Br J Dermatol.* 1989;120:581–584.

Dichi I, Frenhane P, Dichi JB, et al. Comparison of omega-3 fatty acids and sulfasalazine in ulcerative colitis. *Nutrition.* 2000;16(2):87–94.

Dietary supplementation with n-3 polyunsaturated fatty acids and vitamin E after myocardial infarction: Results of the GISSI-Prevenzione trial. *Lancet.* 1999;354:447–455.

Dillon JJ. Fish oil therapy for IgA nephropathy: Efficacy and interstudy variability. *J Am Soc Nephrol.* 1997;8(11):1739–1744.

Djousse L, Pankow JS, Eckfeldt JH, et al. Relation between dietary linolenic acid and coronary artery disease in the National Heart, Lung, and Blood Institute Family Heart Study. *Am J Clin Nutr.* 2001;74(5):612–619.

Dolecek TA. Epidemiological evidence of relationships between dietary polyunsaturated fatty acids and mortality in the multiple risk factor intervention trial. *Proc Soc Exp Biol Med.* 1992;200(2):177–182.

Donadio JV. The emerging role of omega-3 polyunsaturated fatty acids in the management of patients with IgA nephropathy. *J Ren Nutr.* 2001;11(3):122–128.

Donadio JV. Use of fish oil to treat patients with immunoglobulin A nephropathy. *Am J Clin Nutr.* 2000;71(1; suppl):373S–375S.

Donadio JV, Bergstralh EJ, Offord KP, Spencer DC, Holley KE. A controlled trial of fish oil in IgA nephropathy. *N Engl J Med.* 1994;331:1194–1199.

Dooper MM, Wassink L, M'Rabet L, Graus YM. The modulatory effects of prostaglandin-E on cytokine production by human peripheral blood mononuclear cells are independent of the prostaglandin subtype. *Immunol.* 2002;107:152–159.

Drazen JM. COX-2 inhibitors: A lesson in unexpected problems. *N Engl J Med.* 2005; 352:1131–1132.

Dry J, Vincent D. Effect of a fish oil diet on asthma: Results of a 1-year double-blind study. *Int Arch Allergy Appl Immunol.* 1991;95(2–3):156–157.

Duncan BB, Schmidt MI, Pankow JS, et al. Low-grade systemic inflammation and the development of type 2 diabetes: The Atherosclerosis Risk in Communities Study. *Diabetes.* 2003;52:1799–1805.

Durrington PN, Bhatnagar D, Mackness MI, et al. An omega-3 polyunsaturated fatty acid concentrate administered for one year decreased triglycerides in simvastatin treated patients with coronary heart disease and persisting hypertriglyceridaemia. *Heart.* 2001; 85:544–548.

Dyerberg J, Bang HO. A hypothesis on the development of acute myocardial infarction in Greenlanders. *Scand J Clin Lab Invest Suppl.* 1982;161:7–13.

Dyerberg J, Bang HO, Stofferson E, Moncada S, Vane JR. Eicosapentaenoic acid and prevention of thrombosis and atherosclerosis. *Lancet.* 1978;2:117–119.

Ebbesson SO, Kennish J, Ebbesson L, Go O, Yeh J. Diabetes is related to fatty acid imbalance in Eskimos. *Int J Circumpolar Health.* 1999;58:108–119.

Ebbesson SO, Schraer C, Nobmann ED, Ebbesson LO. Lipoprotein profiles in Alaskan Siberian Yupik Eskimos. *Arctic Med Res.* 1996;55:165–173.

Ebel JG, Jr., Eckerlin RH, Maylin GA, Gutenmann WH, Lisk DJ. Polychlorinated biphenyls and p,p'-DDE in encapsulated fish oil supplements. *Nutr Rept Intl.* 1987; 36:413–417.

Eid A, Berry EM. The relationship between dietary fat, adipose tissue composition, and neoplasms of the breast. *Nutr Cancer.* 1988;11:173–177.

Ellis JL. Cardiovascular disease risk factors in Native Americans: A literature review. *Am J Prev Med.* 1994;10:295–307.

Emken EA, Adlof RO, Gulley RM. Dietary linoleic acid influences desaturation and acylation of deuterium-labeled linoleic and linolenic acids in young adult males. *Biochim Biophys Acta.* 1994;1213:277–288.

Erickson KL. Dietary fat, breast cancer, and nonspecific immunity. *Nutr Rev.* 1998; 56:S99–S105.

Eritsland J, Arnesen H, Gronseth K, Fjeld NB, Abdelnoor M. Effect of dietary supplementation with n-3 fatty acids on coronary artery bypass graft patency. *Am J Cardiol.* 1996;77:31–36.

Erlinger TP, Platz EA, Rifai N, Helzlsouer KJ. C-Reactive protein and the risk of incident colorectal cancer. *JAMA.* 2004;291:585–590.

Escobar SO, Achenbach R, Iannantuono R, et al. Topical fish oil in psoriasis: A controlled and blind study. *Clin Exp Dermatol.* 1992;17(3):159–162.

Escrich E, Solanas M, Segura R. Experimental diets for the study of lipid influence on the induced mammary carcinoma in rats: I-diet definition. *In Vivo.* 1994;8:1099–1106.

Etkind PR. Dietary effects on gene expression in mammary tumorigenesis. *Adv Exp Med Biol.* 1995;375:75–83.

Ewertz M, Gill C. Dietary factors and breast-cancer risk in Denmark. *Int J Cancer.* 1990;46:779–784.

Farkouh ME, Kirshner H, Harrington RA, et al. Comparison of lumiracoxib with naproxen and ibuprofen in the Therapeutic Arthritis Research and Gastrointestinal Event Trial (TARGET), cardiovascular outcomes: Randomised controlled trial. *Lancet.* 2004;364: 675–684.

Farmer A, Montori V, Dinneen S, Clar C. Fish oil in people with type 2 diabetes mellitus. *Cochrane Database Syst Rev.* 2004;(1):CD003205.

Fay MP, Freedman LS, Clifford CK, Midthune DN. Effect of different types and amounts of fat on the development of mammary tumors in rodents: A review. *Cancer Res.* 1997;57:3979–3988.

Fearon KC, Von Meyenfeldt MF, Moses AG, et al. Effect of a protein and energy dense n-3 fatty acid enriched oral supplement on loss of weight and lean tissue in cancer cachexia: A randomised double blind trial. *Gut.* 2003;52(10):1479–1486.

Fenton WS, Dickerson F, Boronow J, et al. A placebo-controlled trial of omega-3 fatty acid (ethyl eicosapentaenoic acid) supplementation for residual symptoms and cognitive impairment in schizophrenia. *Am J Psychiatry.* 2001;158(12):2071–2074.

Fernandes G, Venkatraman JT. Possible mechanisms through which dietary lipids, calorie restriction, and exercise modulate breast cancer. In: Jacobs MM, ed. *Exercise, Calories, Fat, and Cancer.* New York: Plenum Press; 1992:185–201.

FitzGerald GA. COX-2 and beyond: Approaches to prostaglandin inhibition in human disease. *Nat Rev Drug Discov.* 2003;2:879–890.

FitzGerald GA, Patrono C. The coxibs, selective inhibitors of cyclooxygenase-2. *N Engl J Med.* 2001;345:433–442.

Flaten H, Hostmark AT, Kierulf P, et al. Fish-oil concentrate: Effects on variables related to cardiovascular disease. *Am J Clin Nutr.* 1990;52:300–306.

Fortin PR, Lew RA, Liang MH, et al. Validation of a meta-analysis: The effects of fish oil in rheumatoid arthritis. *J Clin Epidemiol.* 1995;48(11):1379–1390.

Foulon T, Richard MJ, Payen N, et al. Effects of fish oil fatty acids on plasma lipids and lipoproteins and oxidant-antioxidant imbalance in healthy subjects. *Scand J Clin Lab Invest.* 1999;59:239–248.

French MA, Parrot AM, Kielo ES, et al. Polyunsaturated fat in the diet may improve intestinal function in patients with CD. *Biochim Biophys Acta.* 1997;1360:262–270.

Friedberg CE, Janssen MJ, Heine RJ, Grobbee DE. Fish oil and glycemic control in diabetes: A meta-analysis. *Diabetes Care.* 1998;21:494–500.

Fritsche KL, Johnston PV. Rapid autooxidation of fish oil in diets without added antioxidants. *J Nutr.* April 1988; 118(4):425–426.

Gaard M, Tretli S, Loken EB. Dietary fat and the risk of breast cancer: A prospective study of 25,892 Norwegian women. *Int J Cancer.* 1995;63:13–17.

Gabor H, Abraham S. Effect of dietary menhaden oil on tumor cell loss and the accumulation of mass of a transplantable mammary adenocarcinoma in BALB/c mice. *J Natl Cancer Inst.* 1986;75:1223–1229.

Galli C, Butrum R. Dietary omega-3 fatty acids and cancer: An overview. *World Rev Nutr Diet.* 1991;66:446–461.

Galli C, Simopoulos AP, Tremoli E, eds. Effects of fatty acids and lipids in health and disease. Proceedings of the 1st International Congress of the International Society for the Study of Fatty Acids and Lipids (ISSFAL). Lugano, Switzerland, June 30–July 3, 1993. *World Rev Nutr Diet* 1994;76:1–152.

Gapinski JP, VanRuiswyk JV, Heudebert GR, et al. Preventing restenosis with fish oils following coronary angioplasty: A meta-analysis. *Arch Intern Med.* 1993;153(13): 1595–1601.

Garcia-Closas R, Serra-Majem L, Segura R. Fish consumption, omega-3 fatty acids and the Mediterranean diet. *Eur J Clin Nutr.* September 1993;47(suppl 1):S85–S90.

Gaziano JM, Hennekens CH, O'Donnell CJ, Breslow JL, Buring JE. Fasting triglyceride, high-density lipoprotein and risk of myocardial infarction. *Circulation.* 1997;96:2520–2525.

Gerber, M. Olive oil, monounsaturated fatty acids, and cancer. *Cancer Lett.* 1997; 114:91–92.

German NS, Johanning GL. Eicosapentaenoic acid and epidermal growth factor modulation of human breast cancer cell adhesion. *Cancer Lett.* 1997;118:95–100.

Geusens P, Wouters C, Nijs J, et al. Long-term effect of omega-3 fatty acid supplementation in active rheumatoid arthritis: A 12-month, double-blind, controlled study. *Arthritis Rheum.* 1994;37(6):824–829.

Giani E, Masi I, Galli I. Heated fat, vitamin E and vascualar eicosanoids. *Lipids.* 1985; 20:439.

Gillum RF, Mussolino ME, Madans JH. The relationship between fish consumption and stroke incidence: The NHANES I epidemiologic follow-up study (National Health and Nutrition Examination Survey). *Arch Intern Med.* 1996;156(5):537–542.

Giovannucci E, Rimm EB, Colditz GA, et al. A prospective study of dietary fat and risk of prostate cancer [see comments]. *J Natl Cancer Inst.* 1993;85:1571–1579.

Glaspy J. Nutritional, hormonal, and environmental mechanisms in breast tumorigenesis. In Heber D, Kritchevsky D, eds. *Dietary Fats, Lipids, Hormones, and Tumorigenesis.* New York: Plenum Press; 1996:27–40.

Glaum M, Metzelthin E, Junker S, et al. [Comparative effect of oral fat loads with saturated, omega-6 and omega- 3 fatty acids before and after fish oil capsule therapy in healthy probands]. *Klin Wochenschr.* 1990;68(suppl 22):103–105. [Article in German]

Godley PA. Essential fatty acid consumption and risk of breast cancer. *Breast Cancer Res Treat.* 1995:35, 91–95.

Gogos CA, Ginopoulos P, Salsa B, et al. Dietary omega-3 polyunsaturated fatty acids plus vitamin E restore immunodeficiency and prolong survival for severely ill patients with generalized malignancy: A randomized control trial. *Cancer.* 1998;82:395–402.

Gonzalez MJ, Schemmel RA, Gray JI, Dugan L Jr, Sheffield LG, Welsch CW. Effect of dietary fat on growth of MCF-7 and MDA-MB231 human breast carcinomas in athymic nude mice: Relationship between carcinoma growth and lipid peroxidation product levels. *Carcinogenesis.* 1991;12:1231–1235.

Goodwin PJ, Boyd NF. Critical appraisal of the evidence that dietary fat intake is related to breast cancer risk in humans. *J Natl Cancer Inst.* 1987;79:473–485.

Gordon DJ. Factors affecting high-density lipoproteins. *Endocrinol Metab Clin North Am.* 1998;27:699–709.

Graham S, Hellmann R, Marshall J, et al. Nutritional epidemiology of postmenopausal breast cancer in western New York. *Am J Epidemiol.* 1991;134:552–566.

Graham S, Marshall J, Mettlin C, Rzepka T, Nemoto T, Byers T. Diet in the epidemiology of breast cancer. *Am J Epidemiol.* 1982;116:68–75.

Graham S, Zielezny M, Marshall J, et al. Diet in the epidemiology of postmenopausal breast cancer in the New York State cohort. *Am J Epidemiol.* 1992;136:1327–1337.

Greenfield SM, Green AT, Teare JP, et al. A randomized controlled study of evening primrose oil and fish oil in ulcerative colitis. *Aliment Pharmacol Ther.* 1993;7(2):159–166.

Greenlund J, Valdez R, Casper M. Prevalence and correlates of the insulin resistance syndrome among Native Americans. *Diabetes Care.* 1999;22:441–447.

Greenwald P. Role of dietary fat in the causation of breast cancer: Point. *Cancer Epidemiol Biomarkers Prev.* 1999;8:3–7.

Greenwald P, Sherwood K, McDonald S. Fat, caloric intake, and obesity: Lifestyle risk factors for breast cancer. *J Am Diet Assoc.* 1997;97(suppl):S24–S30.

Grimminger F, Mayser P, Papavassilis C, et al. A double-blind, randomized, placebo-controlled trial of n-3 fatty acid based lipid infusion in acute, extended guttate psoriasis: Rapid improvement of clinical manifestations and changes in neutrophil leukotriene profile. *Clin Invest.* 1993;71(8):634–643.

Grimsgaard S, Bonaa KH, Hansen JB, et al. Highly purified eicosapentaenoic acid and docosahexaenoic acid in humans have similar triacylglycerol-lowering effects but divergent effects on serum fatty acids. *Am J Clin Nutr.* 1997;66(3):649–659.

Grundy SM. N-3 fatty acids: Priority for post-myocardial infarction clinical trials [editorial]. *Circulation.* 2003;107:1834–1836.

Guallar E, Aro A, Jimenez FJ, et al. Omega-3 fatty acids in adipose tissue and risk of myocardial infarction: The EURAMIC Study. *Arterioscler Thromb Vasc Biol.* 1999;19:1111–1118.

Gupta AK, Ellis CN, Goldfarb MT, et al. The role of fish oil in psoriasis: A randomized, double-blind, placebo-controlled study to evaluate the effect of fish oil and topical corticosteroid therapy in psoriasis. *Int J Dermatol.* 1990;29(8):591–595.

Gupta AK, Ellis CN, Tellner DC, et al. Double-blind, placebo-controlled study to evaluate the efficacy of fish oil and low-dose UVB in the treatment of psoriasis. *Br J Dermatol.* 1989;120(6):801–807.

Halliwell B, Gutteridge JM. *Free radicals in biology and medicine.* 3rd ed. New York: Oxford University Press; 1999.

Hansen J, Pedersen H, Mulvad G. Fatty acids and antioxidants in the Inuit diet: Their role in ischemic heart disease (IHD) and possible interactions with other dietary factors. A review. *Arctic Med Res.* 1994;53:4–17.

Hansen JM, Lokkegaard H, Hoy CE, et al. No effect of dietary fish oil on renal hemodynamics, tubular function, and renal functional reserve in long-term renal transplant recipients. *J Am Soc Nephrol.* 1995;5:1434–1440.

Harel Z, Biro FM, Kottenhahn RK, et al. Supplementation with omega-3 polyunsaturated fatty acids in the management of dysmenorrhea in adolescents. *Am J Obstet Gynecol.* 1996;174:1335–1338.

Harris W. The omega-3 index: A new risk factor for death from coronary heart disease? *Prev Med.* 2004;39:212–220.

Harris WS. Fish oils and plasma lipid and lipoprotein metabolism in humans: A critical review. *J Lipid Res.* 1989;30:785–807.

Harris WS. N-3 fatty acids and serum lipoproteins: Human studies. *Am J Clin Nutr* 1997;65(suppl):1645S–1654S.

Harris WS, Dujovne CA, Zucker M, et al. Effects of a low saturated fat, low cholesterol fish oil supplement in hypertriglyceridemic patients: A placebo-controlled trial. *Ann Intern Med.* 1988;109:465–470.

Harris WS, Ginsberg HN, Arunakul N, et al. Safety and efficacy of Omacor in severe hypertriglyceridemia. *J Cardiovasc Risk.* 1997;4:385–391.

Harris WS, Zucker ML, Dujovne CA. Omega-3 fatty acids in hypertriglyceridemic patients: Triglycerides vs. methyl esters. Am J Clin Nutr 1988; 48:992–997.

Hashimoto M, Hossain S, Shimada T, et al. Docosahexaenoic acid provides protection from impairment of learning ability in Alzheimer's disease model rats. *J Neurochem.* 2002;81:1084–1091.

Hatala MA, Rayburn J, Rose DP. Comparison of linoleic acid and eicosapentaenoic acid incorporation into human breast cancer cells. *Lipids.* 1994;29:831–837.

Hawthorne AB, Daneshmend TK, Hawkey CJ, et al. Fish oil in ulcerative colitis: Final results of a controlled clinical trial [abstract]. *Gastroenterology.* 1990;98(5; part 2):A174.

Hawthorne AB, Daneshmend TK, Hawkey CJ, et al. Treatment of ulcerative colitis with fish oil supplementation: A prospective 12-month randomised controlled trial. *Gut.* 1992;33(7):922–928.

Heber D. Interrelationships of high fat diets, obesity, hormones, and cancer. In: Heber D,

Kritchevsky, eds. *Dietary Fats, Lipids, Hormones, and Tumorigenesis.* New York: Plenum Press; 1996:206–233.

Hebert JR, Rosen A. Nutritional, socioeconomic, and reproductive factors in relation to female breast cancer mortality: Findings from a cross-national study. *Cancer Detect Prev.* 1996;20:234–244.

Helland IB, Saugstad OD, Smith L, et al. Similar effects on infants of n-3 and n-6 fatty acids supplementation to pregnant and lactating women. *Pediatrics.* 2001;108(5):E82.

Helland IB, Smith L, Saarem K, Saugstad OD, Drevon CA. Maternal supplementation with very-long-chain n-3 fatty acids during pregnancy and lactation augments children's IQ at 4 years of age. *Pediatrics.* 2003;111(1):E39–E44.

Henderson WR. Omega-3 supplementation in CF [abstract]. *Proceedings of the 6th North American Cystic Fibrosis Conference.* 1992:S21–S22.

Henderson WR Jr, Astley SJ, McCready MM, et al. Oral absorption of omega-3 fatty acids in patients with cystic fibrosis who have pancreatic insufficiency and in healthy control subjects. *J Pediatr.* 1994;124(3):400–408.

Henderson WR Jr, Astley SJ, Ramsey BW. Liver function in patients with cystic fibrosis ingesting fish oil. *J Pediatr.* 1994;125(3):504–505.

Hendra TJ, Britton ME, Roper DR, et al. Effects of fish oil supplements in NIDDM subjects. Controlled study. *Diabetes Care.* 1990;13:821–829.

Henneicke-von Zepelin HH, Mrowietz U, Farber L, et al. Highly purified omega-3 polyunsaturated fatty acids for topical treatment of psoriasis: Results of a double-blind, placebo-controlled multicentre study. *Br J Dermatol.* 1993;129(6):713–717.

Hermann M, Krum H, Ruschitzka F. To the heart of the matter: Coxibs, smoking, and cardiovascular risk. *Circulation.* 2005;112:941–945.

Heude B, Ducimetiere P, Berr C. Cognitive decline and fatty acid composition of erythrocyte membranes: The EVA study. *Am J Clin Nutr.* 2003;77:803–808.

Hibbeln JR. Seafood consumption, the DHA content of mothers' milk and prevalence rates of postpartum depression: A cross-national, ecological analysis. *J Affect Disord.* 2002;69(1–3):15–29.

Hibbeln JR, Salem N, Jr. Dietary polyunsaturated fatty acids and depression: When cholesterol does not satisfy. *Am J Clin Nut.* 1995;62(1):1–9.

Hirayama T. Epidemiology of breast cancer with special reference to the role of diet. *Prev Med.* 1978;7:173–195.

Hirohata T, Nomura AMY, Hankin JH, Kolonel LN, Lee J. An epidemiologic study on the association between diet and breast cancer. *J Natl Cancer Inst.* 1987;78:595–600.

Hirose K, Tajima K, Hamajima N, et al. A large-scale, hospital-based case-control study of risk factors of breast cancer according to menopausal status. *Jpn J Cancer Res.* 1995; 86:146–154.

Hirose M, Masuda A, Ito N, Kamano K, Okuyama H. Effects of dietary perilla oil, soybean oil and safflower oil on 7,12-dimethylbenz[a]anthracene (DMBA) and 1,2-dimethyl-carcinogenesis in female SD rats. *Carcinogenesis.* 1990;11:731–735.

Hislop TG, Coldman AJ, Elwood JM, Brauer G, Kan L. Childhood and recent eating patterns and risk of breast cancer. *Cancer Detect Prev.* 1986;9:47–58.

Hites RA, Foran JA, Carpenter DO, Hamilton MC, Knuth BA, Schwager SJ. Global assessment of organic contaminants in farmed salmon. *Science* 2004;303:226–229.

Hodge L, Salome CM, Peat JK, Haby MM, Xuan W, Woolcock AJ. Consumption of oil fish and childhood asthma risk. *Med J Aust.* 1996;164(3):135–136.

Hodgins S. *Health and What Affects It in Nunavik: How Is the Situation Changing?* Kuujjuaq, Canada: Nunavik Regional Board of Health and Social Services; 1997:7–18.

Hoffman DR, Birch EE, Birch DG, et al. Effects of supplementation with omega-3 long-chain polyunsaturated fatty acids on retinal and cortical development in premature infants. *Am J Clin Nutr.* 1993;57(suppl):807S–812S.

Hojo N, Fukushima T, Isobe A, et al. Effect of serum fatty acid composition on coronary atherosclerosis in Japan. *Int J Cardiol.* 1998;66:31–38.

Holm T, Andreassen AK, Aukrust P, et al. Omega-3 fatty acids improve blood pressure control and preserve renal function in hypertensive heart transplant recipients. *Eur Heart J.* 2001;22(5):428–436.

Holmberg L, Ohlander EM, Byers T, et al. Diet and breast cancer risk: Results from a population-based, case-control study in Sweden. *Arch Intern Med.* 1994;154:1805–1811.

Holmes MD, Hunter DJ, Colditz GA, et al. Association of dietary intake of fat and fatty acids with risk of breast cancer. *JAMA.* 1999;281:914–920.

Holub BJ, Bakker DJ, Skeaff CM. Alterations in molecular species of cholesterol esters formed via plasma lecithin-cholesterol acyltransferase in human subjects consuming fish oil. *Atherosclerosis.* 1987;66:11–18.

Homan van der Heide JJ, Bilo HJ, Donker AJ, et al. Dietary supplementation with fish oil modifies renal reserve filtration capacity in postoperative, cyclosporin A-treated renal transplant recipients. *Transpl Int.* 1990;3(3):171–175.

Homan van der Heide JJ, Bilo HJ, Donker AJ, et al. The effects of dietary supplementation with fish oil on renal function and the course of early postoperative rejection episodes in cyclosporine-treated renal transplant recipients. *Transplantation.* 1992;54(2):257–263.

Homan van der Heide JJ, Bilo HJ, Tegzess AM, et al. Omega-3 polyunsaturated fatty acids improve renal function in renal transplant recipients treated with cyclosporin-A [abstract]. *Kidney Int.* 1989;35:516A.

Hooper L, Summerbell CD, Higgins JP, et al. Dietary fat intake and prevention of cardiovascular disease: Systematic review. *BMJ.* 2001; 322:757–763.

Horrobin DF. Fatty acids, aggression and impulsivity. In: Maes M, Coccaro E, eds. *Neurobiology and Clinical Views on Aggression and Impulsivity.* New York: John Wiley & Sons; 1998.

Horrobin DF. Fatty acids and nervous system disorders. In: Kremer JM, ed. *Medicinal Fatty Acids in Inflammation.* Basel: Bierkhauser; 1998:65–71.

Horrobin DF. Low prevalence of coronary heart disease (CHD), psoriasis, asthma and rheumatoid arthritis in Eskimos: Are they caused by high dietary intake of eicosapentaenoic acid (EPA), a genetic variation of essential fatty acid (EFA) metabolism or a combination of both? *Med Hypotheses.* 1987;22:421–428.

Horrobin DF. Omega-3 fatty acid for schizophrenia. *Am J Psychiatry.* 2003;160(1):188–189.

Horrobin DF. Schizophrenia as a membrane lipid disorder which is expressed throughout the body. *Prostaglandins Leukot Essen Fatty Acids.* 1996; 55(1,2):3–7.

Howe GR, Friedenreich CM, Jain M, Miller AB. A cohort study of fat intake and risk of breast cancer. *J Natl Cancer Inst.* 1991;83:336–340.

Howe GR, Hirohata T, Hislop TG, et al. Dietary factors and risk of breast cancer: Combined analysis of 12 case-control studies. *J Natl Cancer Inst.* 1990;82:561–569.

Howe PR. Dietary fats and hypertension: Focus on fish oil. *Ann N Y Acad Sci.* 1997; 827:339–352.

Hu FB, Bronner L, Willett WC, et al. Fish and omega-3 fatty acid intake and risk of coronary heart disease in women. *JAMA.* 2002;287:1815–1821.

Hu FB, Cho E, Rexrode KM, Albert CM, Manson JE. Fish and long-chain omega-3 fatty acid intake and risk of coronary heart disease and total mortality in diabetic women. *Circulation.* 2003;107(14):1852–1857.

Hu FB, Stampfer MJ, Manson JE, et al. Dietary intake of alpha-linolenic acid and risk of fatal ischemic heart disease among women. *Am J Clin Nutr.* 1999;69(5):890–897.

Hubbard NE, Lim D, Erickson KL. Alteration of murine mammary tumorigenesis by dietary enrichment with n-3 fatty acids in fish oil. *Cancer Lett.* 1998;124:1–7.

Hunter DJ. Role of dietary fat in the causation of breast cancer: Counterpoint. *Cancer Epidemiol Biomarkers Prev.* 1999;8:9–13.

Hunter DJ, Spiegelman D, Adami H-O, et al. Cohort studies of fat intake and the risk of breast cancer: A pooled analysis. *New Engl J Med.* 1996;334:356–361.

Hunter DJ, Spiegelman D, Willett W. Dietary fat and breast cancer [letter; comment]. *J Natl Cancer Inst.* 1998;90:1303–1306.

Hursting SD, Thornquist M, Henderson MM. Types of dietary fat and the incidence of cancer at five sites. *Prev Med.* 1990;19:242–253.

Hussey HJ, Tisdale MJ. Effect of a cachectic factor on carbohydrate metabolism and attenuation by eicosapentaenoic acid. *Br J Cancer.* 1999;80:1231–1235.

Iigo M, Ishikawa C, Kuhara T, et al. Inhibitory effects of oleic and docosahexaenoic acids on lung metastasis by colon-carcinoma-26 cells are associated with reduced matrix metalloproteinase-2 and -9 activities. *Int J Cancer.* 1997;73:607–612.

Iigo M, Nakagawa T, Ishikawa C, et al. Inhibitory effects of docosahexaenoic acid on colon carcinoma 26 metastasis to the lung. *Br J Cancer.* 1997;75(5):650–655.

Ingram DM, Nottage E, Roberts T. The role of diet in the development of breast cancer: A case-control study of patients with breast cancer, benign epithelial hyperplasia and fibrocystic disease of the breast. *Br J Cancer.* 1991;64:187–191.

Ip C. Controversial issues of dietary fat and experimental mammary carcinogenesis. *Prev Med.* 1993;22:728–737.

Ip C. Review of the effects of trans fatty acids, oleic acid, n-3 polyunsaturated fatty acids, and conjugated linoleic acid on mammary carcinogenesis in mammals. *Am J Clin Nutr.* 1997;66(suppl):1523S–1529S.

Ip C, Carter CA, Ip MM. Requirement of essential fatty acid for mammary tumorigenesis in the rat. *Cancer Res.* 1985;45:1997–2001.

Iscovich JM, Iscovich RB, Howe G, Shiboski S, Kaldor JM. A case-control study of diet and breast cancer in Argentina. *Int J Cancer.* 1989;44:770–776.

Iso H, Rexrode KM, Stampfer MJ, et al. Intake of fish and omega-3 fatty acids and risk of stroke in women. *JAMA.* 2001;285(3):304–312.

Jacobs DRJ, Mebane IL, Bangdiwala SI, Criqui MH, Tyroler HA. High-density lipoprotein cholesterol as a predictor of cardiovascular disease mortality in men and women: The follow-up study of the Lipid Research Clinics Prevalence Study. *Am J Epidemiol.* 1990; 131:32–47.

Jacobs MN, Santillo D, Johnston PA, Wyatt CL, French MC. Organochlorine residues in fish oil dietary supplements: Comparison with industrial grade oils. *Chemosphere.* 1998; 37:1709.

Jain M, Miller AB. Tumor characteristics and survival of breast cancer patients in relation to premorbid diet and body size. *Breast Cancer Res Treat.* 1997;42:43–55.

James MJ, Cleland LG. Dietary n-3 fatty acids and therapy for rheumatoid arthritis. *Semin Arthritis Rheum.* 1997;27:85–97.

Johansen O, Brekke M, Seljeflot I, et al. N-3 fatty acids do not prevent restenosis after coronary angioplasty: Results from the CART Study. Coronary Angioplasty Restenosis Trial. *J Am Coll Cardiol.* 1999;33(6):1619–1626.

Jones DY, Schatzkin A, Green SB, et al. Dietary fat and breast cancer in the National Health and Nutrition Examination Survey I epidemiologic follow-up study. *J Natl Cancer Inst.* 1987;79:465–471.

Jones SC. Relative thromboembolic risks associated with COX-2 inhibitors. *Ann Pharmacother.* 2005;39:1249–1259.

Joy CB, Mumby-Croft R, Joy LA. Polyunsaturated fatty acid (fish or evening primrose oil) for schizophrenia. *Cochrane Database Syst Rev.* 2000;(2):CD001257.

Juni P, Reichenbach S, Egger M. COX-2 inhibitors, traditional NSAIDs, and the heart. *BMJ.* 2005;330:1342–1343.

Jurkowski JJ, Cave W Jr. Dietary effects of menhaden oil on growth and membrane lipid composition of rat mammary tumors. *J Natl Cancer Inst.* 1983;74:1145–1150.

Kaizer L, Boyd NF, Kriukov V, Tritchler D. Fish consumption and breast cancer risk: An ecological study. *Nutr Cancer.* 1989;12:61–68.

Kalmijn S, Launer LJ, Ott A, Witteman JC, Hofman A, Breteler MM. Dietary fat intake and the risk of incident dementia in the Rotterdam Study. *Ann Neurol.* 1997;42:776–782.

Kannel WB. Fifty years of Framingham Study contributions to understanding hypertension. *J Hum Hypertens.* 2000;14:83–90.

Karmali RA. N-3 fatty acids and cancer. *J Intern Med.* 1989;225:197-200.

Kato I, Miura S, Kasumi F, et al. A case-control study of breast cancer among Japanese women: With special reference to family history and reproductive and dietary factors. *Breast Cancer Res Treat.* 1992;24:51–59.

Katsouyanni K, Trichopoulou A, Stuver S, et al. The association of fat and other macronutrients with breast cancer: A case-control study from Greece. *Br J Cancer.* 1994;70: 537–541.

Katsouyanni K, Willett W, Trichopoulos D, et al. Risk of breast cancer among Greek women in relation to nutrient intake. *Cancer.* 1988;61:181–185.

Katz DP, Manner T, Furst P, et al. The use of an intravenous fish oil emulsion enriched with omega-3 fatty acids in patients with cystic fibrosis. *Nutrition.* 1996;12(5):334–339.

Keli SO, Feskens EJ, Kromhout D. Fish consumption and risk of stroke: The Zutphen Study. *Stroke.* 1994;25(2):328–332.

Kelsey JL, Bernstein L. Epidemiology and prevention of breast cancer. *Annu Rev Public Health.* 1996;17:47–67.

Kestin M, Clifton P, Belling GB, Nestel PJ. N-3 fatty acids of marine origin lower systolic blood pressure and triglycerides but raise LDL cholesterol compared with n-3 and n-6 fatty acids from plants. *Am J Clin Nutr.* 1990;51:1028–1034.

Kim YI. Can fish oil maintain Crohn's disease in remission? *Nutr Rev.* 1996;54(8):248–252.

Kinrys G. Hypomania associated with omega-3 fatty acids. *Arch Gen Psychiatry.* 2000;57(7):715–716.

Kjeldsen-Kragh J, Lund JA, Riise T, et al. Dietary omega-3 fatty acid supplementation and naproxen treatment in patients with rheumatoid arthritis. *J Rheumatol.* 1992; 19(10):1531–1536.

Klein JR, Litt IF. Epidemiology of adolescent dysmenorrhea. *Pediatrics.* 1981;68:661–664.

Klein V, Chajes V, Germain E, et al. Low alpha-linolenic acid content of adipose breast tissue is associated with an increased risk of breast cancer. *Eur J Cancer.* 2000;36(3): 335–340.

Knapp HR. Dietary fatty acids in human thrombosis and hemostasis. *Am J Clin Nutr.* 1997;65(5; suppl):1687S–1698S.

Knapp HR, FitzGerald GA. The antihypertensive effects of fish oil: A controlled study of polyunsaturated fatty acid supplements in essential hypertension. *N Engl J Med.* 1989;320(16):1037–1043.

Knekt P, Albanes D, Seppanen R, et al. Dietary fat and risk of breast cancer. *Am J Clin Nutr.* 1990;52:903–908.

Kohlmeier L, Mendez M. Controversies surrounding diet and breast cancer. *Proc Nutr Soc.* 1997;56:369–382.

Kohlmeier L, Simonsen N, van't Veer P, et al. Adipose tissue trans fatty acids and breast cancer in the Eurpoean community multicenter study on antioxidants, myocardial infarction, and breast cancer. *Cancer Epidemiol Biomarkers Prev.* 1997;6:705–710.

Kojima T, Ternao T, Tanabe E, et al. Effect of highly purified eicosapentaenoic acid on psoriasis. *J Am Acad Dermatol.* 1989;21:150–151.

Kojima T, Terano T, Tanabe E, et al. Long-term administration of highly purified eicosapentaenoic acid provides improvement of psoriasis. *Dermatologica.* 1991;182:225–230.

Konard RJ, Stoller JZ, Gao ZY, Wolf BA. Eicosapentaenoic acid (C20:5) augments glucose-induced insulin secretion from beta-TC3 insulinoma cells. *Pancreas.* October 1996; 13(3):253–258.

Konstam MA, Weir MR, Reicin AS, et al. Cardiovascular thrombotic events in controlled, clinical trials of rofecoxib. *Circulation.* 2001;104:2280–2288.

Konstantinopoulos PA, Lehmann DF. The cardiovascular toxicity of selective and nonselective cyclooxygenase inhibitors: Comparisons, contrasts, and aspirin confounding. *J Clin Pharmacol.* 2005;45:742–750.

Kooijmans-Coutinho MF, Rischen-Vos J, Hermans J, et al. Dietary fish oil in renal transplant recipients treated with cyclosporin-A: No beneficial effects shown. *J Am Soc Nephrol.* 1996;7(3):513–518.

Koretz RL. Maintaining remissions in Crohn's disease: A fat chance to please. *Gastroenterology.* 1997;112(6):2155–2156.

Kort WJ, Weijma IM, Bijma AM, van Schalkwijk WP, Vergroesen AJ, Westbroek DL. Omega-3 fatty acids inhibiting the growth of a transplantable rat mammary adenocarcinoma. *J Natl Cancer Inst.* 1987;79:593–599.

Kremer JM, Bigauoette J, Michalek AV, et al. Effects of manipulation of dietary fatty acids on clinical manifestations of rheumatoid arthritis. *Lancet.* 1985;1(8422):184–187.

Kremer JM, Jubiz W, Michalek A, et al. Fish-oil fatty acid supplementation in active rheumatoid arthritis: A double-blinded, controlled, crossover study. *Ann Intern Med.* 1987;106(4):497–503.

Kremer JM, Lawrence DA, Jubiz W, et al. Dietary fish oil and olive oil supplementation in patients with rheumatoid arthritis: Clinical and immunologic effects. *Arthritis Rheum.* 1990;33:810–820.

Kremer JM, Lawrence DA, Petrillo GF, et al. Effects of high-dose fish oil on rheumatoid arthritis after stopping nonsteroidal antiinflammatory drugs: Clinical and immune correlates. *Arthritis Rheum.* 1995;38:1107–1114.

Kris-Etherton PM, Harris WS, Appel LJ. Fish consumption, fish oil, omega-3 fatty acids, and cardiovascular disease [published correction appears in *Circulation* 2003;107(3): 512]. *Circulation.* 2002;106(21):2747–2757.

Kris-Etherton PM, Taylor DS, Yu-Poth S, et al. Polyunsaturated fatty acids in the food chain in the United States. *Am J Clin Nutr.* 2000;71(suppl):179S–88S.

Kristensen SD, Schmidt EB, Andersen HR, et al. Fish oil in angina pectoris. *Atherosclerosis.* 1987;64(1):13–19.

Kristiansen E, Madsen C, Meyer O, Roswall K, Thorup I. Effects of high-fat diet on incidence of spontaneous tumors in Wistar rats. *Nutr Cancer.* 1993;19:99–110.

Kromann N, Green A. Epidemiological studies in the Upernavik district, Greenland: Incidence of some chronic diseases 1950–1974. *Acta Med Scand.* 1980;208(5):401–406.

Kromhout D, Bloemberg BP, Feskens EJ, et al. Alcohol, fish, fibre and antioxidant vitamins intake do not explain population differences in coronary heart disease mortality. *Int J Epidemiol.* 1996;25(4):753–759.

Kromhout D, Bosschieter EB, de Lezenne Coulander C. The inverse relation between fish consumption and 20-year mortality from coronary heart disease. *N Engl J Med.* 1985;312:1205–1209.

Kromhout D, Menotti A, Bloemberg B, et al. Dietary saturated and trans fatty acids and cholesterol and 25-year mortality from coronary heart disease: The Seven Countries Study. *Prev Med.* 1995;308–315.

Kuenzel U, Bertsch S. Clinical experiences with a standardized commercial fish oil product containing 33.5 percent omega-3 fatty acids: Field trial with 3,958 hyperlipemic patients in general practitioner practice. In: Chandra RK, ed. *Health Effects of Fish and Fish Oils.* New Foundland: ARTS Biomedical Publishers and Distributors; 1989:567–579.

Kuhnlein H, Soueida R, Receveur O. Dietary nutrient profiles of Canadian Baffin Island Inuit by food source, season, and age. *J Am Diet Assoc.* 1996;96:155–162.

Kunz B, Ring J, Braun-Falco O. Eicosapentaenoic acid (EPA) treatment in atopic eczema (AE): A prospective double-blind trial [abstract]. *J Allergy Clin Immunol.* 1989;83:196.

Kurlandsky LE, Bennink MR, Webb PM, et al. The absorption and effect of dietary supplementation with omega-3 fatty acids on serum leukotriene B4 in patients with cystic fibrosis. *Pediatr Pulmonol.* 1994;18(4):211–217.

Kushi LH, Lenart EB, Willett WC. Health implications of Mediterranean diets in light of contemporary knowledge. 2. Meat, wine, fats, and oils. *Am J Clin Nutr.* 1995;61(suppl): 1416S–1427S.

Kushi LH, Sellers TA, Potter JD, et al. Dietary fat and postmenopausal breast cancer. *J Natl Cancer Inst.* 1992;84:1092–1099.

Kyle DJ, Schaefer E, Patton G, Beiser A. Low serum docosahexaenoic acid is a significant risk factor for Alzheimer's dementia. *Lipids.* 1999;34:S245.

Lai PB, Ross JA, Fearon KC, Anderson JD, Carter DC. Cell cycle arrest and induction of apoptosis in pancreatic cancer cells exposed to eicosapentaenoic acid in vitro. *Br J Cancer.* 1996;74(9):1375–1383.

Lamarche B, Tchernof A, Mauriège P, et al. Fasting insulin and apolipoprotein B levels and low-density lipoprotein particle size as risk factors for ischemic heart disease. *JAMA.* 1998;279:1955–1961.

Landa M-C, Frago N, Tres A. Diet and the risk of breast cancer in Spain. *Eur J Cancer Prev.* 1994;3:313–320.

Landgraf R. N-3 fatty acids in diabetes mellitus. In: Frolich JC, von Schacky C, eds. *Fish, Fish Oil and Human Health.* Munich, Germany: W Zuckschwerdt Verlag; 1992:123–134.

Lands WEM. Biochemistry and physiology of eicosanoid precursors in cell membranes. *Eur Heart J.* 2001;3(suppl D):D22–D25.

Lands WEM, Libelt B, Morris A, et al. Maintenance of lower proportions of (n-6) eicosanoid precursors in phospholipids of human plasma in response to added dietary (n-3) fatty acids. *Biochim Biophys Acta.* 1992;1180:147–162.

Langman M. Ulcer complications associated with anti-inflammatory drug use: What is the extent of the disease burden? *Pharmacoepidemiol Drug Saf.* 2001;10(1):13–19.

Lanier AP, Bulkow LR, Ireland B. Cancer in Alaskan Indians, Eskimos, and Aleuts, 1969–83: Implications for etiology and control. *Public Health Rep.* 1989;104:658–664.

Lardinois CL. The role of omega-3 fatty acids on insulin secretion and insulin sensitivity. *Med Hypotheses.* 1987;24:243–248.

Lau CS, Morley KD, Belch JJ. Effects of fish oil supplementation on non-steroidal anti-inflammatory drug requirement in patients with mild rheumatoid arthritis: A double-blind placebo-controlled study. *Br J Rheumatol.* 1993;32:982–989.

Laugharne JD, Mellor JE, Peet M. Fatty acids and schizophrenia. *Lipids.* 1996;31(suppl): S163–S165.

LaVecchia C, Decarli A, Franceschi S, Gentile A, Negri E, Parazzini F. Dietary factors and the risk of breast cancer. *Nutr Cancer.* 1987;10:205–214.

LaVecchia C, Decarli A, Parazzini F, et al. General epidemiology of breast cancer in northern Italy. *Int J Epidemiol.* 1987;16:347–355.

Lawrence R, Sorrell T. Eicosapentaenoic acid in cystic fibrosis: Evidence of a pathogenetic role for leukotriene B4. *Lancet.* 1993;342(8869):465–469.

Lawson LD, Hughes BG. Absorption of eicosapentaenoic acid and docosahexaenoic acid from fish oil triacylglycerols or fish oil ethyl esters co-ingested with a high-fat meal. *Biochem Biophys Res Commun.* 1988;156(2):960–963.

Lazarou J, Pomeranz BH, Corey PN. Incidence of adverse drug reactions in hospitalized patients: A meta-analysis of prospective studies. *JAMA.* 1998;279(15):1200–1205.

Leaf A, Jorgensen MB, Jacobs AK, et al. Do fish oils prevent restenosis after coronary angioplasty? *Circulation.* 1994;90(5):2248–2257.

Leaf A, Kang JX, Xiao YF, Billman GE. Clinical prevention of sudden cardiac death by n-3 polyunsaturated fatty acids and mechanism of prevention of arrhythmias by n-3 fish oils. *Circulation.* 2003;107:2646–2652.

Lee HP, Gourley L, Duffy SW, Esteve J, Lee J, Day NE. Dietary effects on breast cancer risk in Singapore. *Lancet.* 1991;3737:1197–1200.

Lemaitre RN, King IB, Mozaffarian D, Kuller LH, Tracy RP, Siscovick DS. N-3 polyunsaturated fatty acids, fatal ischemic heart disease and non-fatal myocardial infarction in older adults: The Cardiovascular Health Study. *Am J Clin Nutr.* 2002;76:319–325.

Lemieux S, Prud'homme D, Bouchard C, Tremblay A, Després JP. A single threshold value of waist girth identifies normal-weight and overweight subjects with excess visceral adipose tissue. *Am J Clin Nutr.* 1996;64:685–693.

Leng GC, Taylor GS, Lee AJ, Fowkes FG, Horrobin D. Essential fatty acids and cardiovascular disease: The Edinburgh Artery Study. *Vasc Med.* 1999;4:219–226.

Levi F, La Vecchia C, Gulie C, Negri E. Dietary factors and breast cancer risk in Vaud, Switzerland. *Nutr Cancer.* 1993;19:327–335.

Levy BD, Clish CB, Schmidt B, Gronert K, Serhan CN. Lipid mediator class switching during acute inflammation: Signals in resolution. *Nature Immunol.* 2001;2:612–619.

Lhuillery C, Bougnoux P, Groscolas R, Durand G. Time-course study of adipose tissue fatty acid composition during mammary tumor growth in rats with controlled fat intake. *Nutr Cancer.* 1995;24:299–309.

Lim BO, Jolly CA, Zaman K, Fernandes G. Dietary (n-6) and (n-3) fatty acids and energy restriction modulate mesenteric lymph node lymphocyte function in autoimmune-prone (NZB x NZW)F1 mice. *J Nutr.* 2000;130(7):1657–1664.

Lipworth L, Martinez ME, Angell J, Hsieh C-C, Trichopoulos D. Olive oil and human cancer: An assessment of evidence. *Prev Med.* 1997;26:181–190.

Loeschke K, Ueberschaer B, Pietsch A, et al. N-3 fatty acids only delay early relapse of ulcerative colitis in remission. *Dig Dis Sci.* 1996;41(10):2087–2094.

Logan A. Report of the Canadian Hypertension Society's consensus conference on the management of mild hypertension. *Can Med Assoc J.* 1984;131:1053–1057.

London SJ, Sacks FM, Stampfer MJ, et al. Fatty acid composition of the subcutaneous adipose tissue and risk of proliferative benign breast disease and breast cancer. *J Natl Cancer Inst.* 1993;85:785–793.

Lorenz R, Loeschke K. Placebo-controlled trials of omega 3 fatty acids in chronic inflammatory bowel disease. *World Rev Nutr Diet.* 1994;76:143–145.

Lorenz R, Weber PC, Szimnau P, et al. Supplementation with n-3 fatty acids from fish oil in chronic inflammatory bowel disease: A randomized, placebo-controlled, double- blind cross-over trial. *J Intern Med Suppl.* 1989;225(731):225–232.

Lubin JH, Burns PE, Blot WJ, Ziegler RG, Lees AW, Fraumeni JF Jr. Dietary factors and breast cancer risk. *Int J Cancer.* 1981;28:685–689.

Lund E. The research tide ebbs for the dietary fat hypothesis in breast cancer. *Epidemiology.* 1994;5:387–388.

Lund E, Bonaa KH. Reduced breast cancer mortality among fishermen's wives in Norway. *Cancer Causes Control.* 1993;4:283–287.

Lungershausen YK, Abbey M, Nestel PJ, et al. Reduction of blood pressure and plasma triglycerides by omega-3 fatty acids in treated hypertensives. *J Hypertens.* 1994;12(9): 1041.

Luostarinen R, Boberg M, Saldeen T. Fatty acid composition in total phospholipids of human coronary arteries in sudden cardiac death. *Atherosclerosis.* 1993;99:187–193.

Maachi K, Berthoux P, Burgard G, et al. Results of a 1-year randomized controlled trial with omega-3 fatty acid fish oil in renal transplantation under triple immunosuppressive therapy. *Transplant Proc.* 1995;27(1):846–849.

Malik I. JournalScan. *Heart.* 2005;91:847–848

Malik IA, Sharif S, Malik F, Hakimali A, Khan WA, Badruddin SH. Nutritional aspects of mammary carcinogenesis: A case-control study. *J Pak Med Assoc.* 1993;43:118–120.

Mamdani M, Rochon P, Juurlink DM, et al. Effect of selective cyclooxygenase 2 inhibitors and naproxen on short-term risk of acute myocardial infarction in the elderly. *Arch Intern Med.* 2003;163:481–486.

Marangell LB, Zboyan HA, Cress KK, et al. A double-blind placebo-controlled study of decosahaexanoic acid in the treatment of depression. *Inform.* 2000;11:S78.

Marcheselli VL, Hong S, Lukiw WJ, Tian XH, Gronert K, Musto A, Hardy M, Gimenez JM, Chiang N, Serhan CN, Bazan NG. Novel docosanoids inhibit brain ischemia-reperfusion-mediated leukocyte infiltration and pro-inflammatory gene expression. *J Biol Chem.* 2003;278:43807–43817.

Marchioli R, Barzi F, Bomba E, et al. Early protection against sudden death by n-3 polyunsaturated fatty acids after myocardial infarction: Time-course analysis of the results of the gruppo italiano per lo studio della sopravvivenza nell'infarto miocardico (GISSI)-prevenzione. *Circulation.* 2002;105(16):1897–1903.

Maresta A, Balduccelli M, Varani E, et al. Prevention of postcoronary angioplasty restenosis by omega-3 fatty acids: Main results of the Esapent for Prevention of Restenosis Italian Study (ESPRIT). *Am Heart J.* 2002;143(6):E5.

Maroon, JC, Bost, JW. Omega-3 Fatty acids (fish oil) as an anti-inflammatory: an alternative to nonsteroidal anti-inflammatory drugs for discogenic pain. *Surgical Neurology* April 2006;65:326–331.

Marras C, Tanner CM. Epidemiology of Parkinson's disease. In: Watts RL, Koller WC, eds. *Movement Disorders: Neurologic Principles & Practice.* 2nd ed. New York: McGraw-Hill; 2004:177–195.

Marshall JR, Yinsheng Q, Junshi C, Parpia B, Campbell TC. Additional ecological evidence: Lipids and breast cancer mortality among women aged 55 and over in China. *Eur J Cancer.* 1992;28A:1720–1727.

Martin-Moreno JM, Willett WC, Gorgojo L, et al. Dietary fat, olive oil intake and breast cancer risk. *Int J Cancer.* 1994;58:774–780.

Masuev KA. [The effect of polyunsaturated fatty acids of the omega-3 class on the late phase of the allergic reaction in bronchial asthma patients]. *Ter Arkh.* 1997;69(3):31–33. [Article in Russian.]

Mayser P, Mrowietz U, Arenberger P, et al. Omega-3 fatty acid-based lipid infusion in patients with chronic plaque psoriasis: Results of a double-blind, randomized, placebo-controlled, multicenter trial. *J Am Acad Dermatol.* 1998;38:539–547.

McDonald CF, Vecchie L, Pierce RJ, et al. Effect of fish-oil derived omega-3 fatty acid supplements on asthma control [abstract]. *Austral New Zealand J Med.* 1990;20:526.

McGinnis WR. Oxidative stress in autism. *Altern Ther Health Med.* 2004;10(6):22–36.

Mehrotra B, Ronquillo J. Dietary supplementation in hem/onc outpatients at a tertiary care hospital. American Society of Clinical Oncology 38th Annual Meeting, Orlando, Florida, May 18–20, 2002.

Mellor J, Laugharne JD, Peet M. Omega-3 fatty acid supplementation in schizophrenic patients. *Human Psychopharmacol.* 1996;11:39–46.

Miles EA, Allen E, Calder PC. In vitro effects of eicosanoids derived from different 20-carbon fatty acids on production of monocyte-derived cytokines in human whole blood cultures. *Cytokine.* 2002;20:215–223.

Miller AB. An overview of hormone-associated cancers. *Cancer Res.* 1978;38:3985–3990.

Miller AB, Kelly A, Choi NW, et al. A study of diet and breast cancer. *Am J Epidemiol.* 1978;107:499–509.

Mills PK, Beeson L, Phillips RL, Fraser GE. Dietary habits and breast cancer incidence among Seventh-Day Adventists. *Cancer.* 1989;64:582–590.

Ministère de la santé et des services Sociaux du Québec. [*Mortality Surveillance in Quebec, 1992–1996.*] Québec: Gouvernement du Québec, 1998. [In French.]

Mischoulon D, Fava M. Docosahexanoic acid and omega-3 fatty acids in depression. *Psychiatr Clin North Am.* 2000;23(4):785–794.

Mizushima S, Moriguchi EH, Ishikawa P, et al. Fish intake and cardiovascular risk among middle-aged Japanese in Japan and Brazil. *J Cardiovasc Risk.* 1997;4(3):191–199.

Moffat M, Young TK. Nutritional patterns of Inuit in the Keewatin region of Canada. *Arctic Med Res.* 1994;53:298–300.

Montori VM, Farmer A, Wollan PC, et al. Fish oil supplementation in type 2 diabetes: A quantitative systematic review. *Diabetes Care.* 2000;23(9):1407–1415.

Morel DW, DiCorleto PE, Chisolm GM. Endothelial and smooth muscle cells alter low density lipoprotein in vitro by free radical oxidation. *Arteriosclerosis.* 1984;4:357–64.

Mori TA, Bao DQ, Burke V, Puddey IB, Beilin LJ. Docosahexaenoic acid but not eicosapentaenoic acid lowers ambulatory blood pressure and heart rate in humans. *Hypertension.* 1999;34(2):253–260.

Mori TA, Burke V, Puddey IB, et al. Purified eicosapentaenoic and docosahexaenoic acids have differential effects on serum lipids and lipoproteins, LDL particle size, glucose, and insulin in mildly hyperlipidemic men. *Am J Clin Nutr.* 2000;71:1085–1094.

Mori TA, Watts GF, Burke V, et al. Differential effects of eicosapentaenoic acid and docosahexaenoic acid on vascular reactivity of the forearm microcirculation in hyperlipidemic, overweight men. *Circulation.* 2000;102(11):1264–1269.

Morris MC, Evans DA, Bienias JL, et al. Consumption of fish and n-3 fatty acids and risk of incident Alzheimer disease. *Arch Neurol* 2003; 60:940–946.

Morris MC, Manson JE, Rosner B, et al. Fish consumption and cardiovascular disease in the Physicians' Health Study: A prospective study. *Am J Epidemiol.* 1995;142(2): 166–175.

Morris MC, Sacks F, Rosner B. Does fish oil lower blood pressure? A meta-analysis of controlled trials. *Circulation.* 1993;88:523–533.

Morris MC, Taylor JO, Stampfer MJ, et al. The effect of fish oil on blood pressure in mild hypertensive subjects: A randomized crossover trial. *Am J Clin Nutr.* 1993;57(1):59–64.

Muckle G, Ayotte P, Dewailly É, Jacobson SW, Jacobson JL. Determinants of polychlorinated biphenyls and methylmercury exposure in Inuit women of childbearing age. *Environ Health Perspect.* 2001;109(9)957–963.

Mukherjee DM, Nissen SE, Topol EJ. Risk of cardiovascular events associated with selective COX-2 inhibitors. *JAMA.* 2001;286:954–959.

Mukherjee PK, Marcheselli VL, Serhan CN, Bazan NG. Neuroprotectin D1: A docosahexaenoic acid-derived docosatriene protects human retinal pigment epithelial cells from oxidative stress. *Proc Natl Acad Sci USA.* 2004;101:8491–8496.

Munoz SE, Silva RA, Lamarque A, Guzman CA, Eynard AR. Protective capability of dietary Zizyphus mistol seed oil, rich in 18:3, n-3 on the development of two murine mammary gland adenocarcinomas with high or low metastatic potential. *Prostglandins Leukot Essent Fatty Acids.* 1995;53:135–138.

Nagakura T, Matsuda S, Shichijyo K, et al. Dietary supplementation with fish oil rich in omega-3 polyunsaturated fatty acids in children with bronchial asthma. *Eur Respir J.* 2000;16(5):861–865.

Nakamura N, Hamazaki T, Ohta M, et al. Joint effects of HMG-CoA reductase inhibitors and eicosapentaenoic acids on serum lipid profile and plasma fatty acid concentrations in patients with hyperlipidemia. *Int J Clin Lab Res.* 1999;29(1):22–25.

National Institutes of Health. Clinical guidelines on the identification, evaluation and treatment of overweight and obesity in adults: The evidence report. *Obes Res.* 1998; 6(suppl):51S–209S.

Natvig H, Borchgrevink CF, Dedichen J, Owren PA, Schiotz EH, Westlund K. A controlled trial of the effect of linolenic acid on incidence of coronary heart disease: The Norwegian vegetable oil experiment of 1965–66. *Scand J Clin Lab Invest.* 1968;105 (suppl):1–20.

Nemets B, Stahl Z, Belmaker RH. Addition of omega-3 fatty acid to maintenance medication treatment for recurrent unipolar depressive disorder. *Am J Psychiatry.* 2002; 159(3):477–479.

Nestel PJ. Fish oil and cardiovascular disease: Lipids and arterial function. *Am J Clin Nutr.* 2000;71(suppl):228S–231S.

Newcomb PA, Klein R, Klein BEK, et al. Association of dietary and life-style factors with sex hormones in postmenopausal women. *Epidemiology.* 1995;6:318–321.

Nielsen GL, Faarvang KL, Thomsen BS, et al. The effects of dietary supplementation with n-3 polyunsaturated fatty acids in patients with rheumatoid arthritis: A randomized, double blind trial. *Eur J Clin Invest.* 1992;22(10):687–691.

Nilsen DW, Albrektsen G, Landmark K, et al. Effects of a high-dose concentrate of n-3 fatty acids or corn oil introduced early after an acute myocardial infarction on serum triacylglycerol and HDL cholesterol. *Am J Clin Nutr.* 2001;74(1):50–56.

Nixon DW. Cancer, cancer cachexia, and diet: Lessons from clinical research. *Nutrition.* 1996;12(suppl):S52–S56.

Noguchi M, Earashi M, Minami M, Kinoshita K, Miyazaki I. Effects of eicosapentaenoic and docosahexaenoic acid on cell growth and prostaglandin E and leukotriene B production by a human breast cancer cell line (MDA-MB-231). *Oncology.* 1995;52:458–464.

Noguchi M, Minami M, Yagasaki R, et al. Chemoprevention of DMBA-induced mammary carcinogenesis in rats by low-dose EPA and DHA. *Br J Cancer.* 1997;75:348–353.

Noguchi M, Rose DP, Earashi M, Miyazaki I. The role of fatty acids and eicosanoid synthesis inhibitors in breast carcinoma. *Oncology.* 1995;52:265–271.

Nordoy A, Bonaa KH, Sandset PM, et al. Effect of omega-3 fatty acids and simvastatin on hemostatic risk factors and postprandial hyperlipemia in patients with combined hyperlipemia. *Arterioscler Thromb Vasc Biol.* 2000;20(1):259–265.

Nordoy A, Hansen JB, Brox J, et al. Effects of atorvastatin and omega-3 fatty acids on LDL subfractions and postprandial hyperlipemia in patients with combined hyperlipemia. *Nutr Metab Cardiovasc Dis.* 2001;11(1):7–16.

Nordstrom DC, Honkanen VE, Nasu Y, Antila E, Friman C, Konttinen YT. Alpha-linolenic acid in the treatment of rheumatoid arthritis. A double-blind, placebo-controlled and randomized study: Flaxseed vs. safflower seed. *Rheumatol Int.* 1995;14:231–234.

Norrish AE, Skeaff CM, Arribas GL, Sharpe SJ, Jackson RT. Prostate cancer risk and consumption of fish oils: A dietary biomarker-based case-control study. *Br J Cancer.* 1999;81(7):1238–1242.

Novak TE, Babcock TA, Jho DH, Helton WS, Espat NJ. NF-κB inhibition by ω-3 fatty acids modulates LPS-stimulated macrophage TNF-α transcription. *Am J Physiol.* 2003;284:L84–L89.

Nussmeier NA, Whelton AA, Brown MT, et al. Complications of the COX-2 inhibitors parecoxib and valdecoxib after cardiac surgery. *N Engl J Med.* 2005;352(11):1081–1091.

Nutt JG, Wooten GF. Diagnosis and initial management of Parkinson's disease. *N Engl J Med.* 2005. 353(10):1021–1027.

Okamoto M, Mitsunobu F, Ashida K, et al. Effects of dietary supplementation with n-3 fatty acids compared with n-6 fatty acids on bronchial asthma. *Intern Med.* 2000;39(2): 107–111.

Okie, S. Raising the safety bar: The FDA's coxib meeting. *N Engl J Med.* 2005;352: 1283–1285.

Okuda Y, Mizutani M, Ogawa M, et al. Long-term effects of eicosapentaenoic acid on diabetic peripheral neuropathy and serum lipids in patients with type II diabetes mellitus. *J Diabetes Complications.* 1996;10(5):280–287.

Olsen SF, Secher NJ. Low consumption of seafood in early pregnancy as a risk factor for preterm delivery: Prospective cohort study. *BMJ.* 2002;324(7335):447.

Olsen SF, Secher NJ, Tabor A, et al. Randomised clinical trials of fish oil supplementation in high risk pregnancies. Fish Oil Trials in Pregnancy (FOTIP) Team. *BJOG.* 2000; 107(3):382–395.

Olsen SF, Sorensen JD, Secher NJ, et al. Randomised controlled trial of effect of fish-oil supplementation on pregnancy duration. *Lancet.* 1992;339(8800):1003–1007.

Onwude JL, Lilford RJ, Hjartardottir H, et al. A randomised double-blind placebo-controlled trial of fish oil in high risk pregnancy. *BJOG.* 1995;102(2):95–100.

Oomen CM, Feskens EJM, Rasanen L, et al. Fish consumption and coronary heart disease mortality in Finland, Italy, and the Netherlands. *Am J Epidemiol.* 2000;151: 999–1006.

Oomen CM, Ocke MC, Feskens EJ, van Erp-Baart MA, Kok FJ, Kromhout D. Association between trans fatty acid intake and 10-year risk of coronary heart disease in the Zutphen Elderly Study: A prospective population-based study. *Lancet.* 2001;357(9258):746–751.

Oomen CM, Ocke MC, Feskens EJ, et al. Alpha-linolenic acid intake is not beneficially associated with 10-year risk of coronary artery disease incidence: The Zutphen Elderly Study. *Am J Clin Nutr.* 2001;74(4):457–463.

Orencia AJ, Daviglus ML, Dyer AR, et al. Fish consumption and stroke in men: 30-year findings of the Chicago Western Electric Study. *Stroke.* 1996;27(2):204–209.

Ott E, Nussmeier NA, Duke PC, et al. Efficacy and safety of the cyclo-oxygenase 2 inhibitors parecoxib and valdecoxib in patients undergoing coronary artery bypass surgery. *J Thorac Cardiovasc Surg.* 2003;125:1481–1492.

Paganelli F, Maixent JM, Duran MJ, Parhizgar R, Pieroni G, Sennoune S. Altered erythrocyte n-3 fatty acids in Mediterranean patients with coronary artery disease. *Int J Cardiol.* 2001;78:27–32.

Pala V, Krogh V, Muti P, et al. Erythrocyte membrane fatty acids and subsequent breast cancer: A prospective Italian study. *J Natl Cancer Inst.* 2001;93:1088–1095.

Palat D, Rudolph D, Rothstein M. A trial of fish oil in asthma [abstract]. *Am Rev Respir Dis.* 1988;137(suppl 4, part 2):329.

Pandalai PK, Pilat MJ, Yamazaki K, Naik H, Pienta KJ. The effects of omega-3 and omega-6 fatty acids on in vitro prostate cancer growth. *Anticancer Res.* 1996;16(2): 815–820.

Parkinson AJ, Cruz AL, Heyward WL, et al. Elevated concentrations of plasma -3 polyunsaturated fatty acids among Alaskan Eskimos. *Am J Clin Nutr.* 1994;59:384–388.

Patrick L, Salik R. The effect of essential fatty acid supplementation on language development and learning skills in autism and Asperger's syndrome. *Autism-Asperger's Digest.* Jan/Feb 2005:36–37.

Pawlosky RJ, Hibbeln JR, Lin Y, et al. Effects of beef- and fish-based diets on the kinetics of n-3 fatty acid metabolism in human subjects. *Am J Clin Nutr.* 2003;77:565–572.

Pawlosky RJ, Hibbeln JR, Novotny JA, Salem NJ. Physiological compartmental analysis of alpha-linolenic acid metabolism in adult humans. *J Lipid Res* 2001; 42:1257–1265.

Peet M, Brind J, Ramchand CN, et al. Two double-blind placebo-controlled pilot studies of eicosapentaenoic acid in the treatment ofschiozophrenia. *Schizophr Res.* 2001;49(3): 243–251.

Peet M, Horrobin DF. A dose-ranging study of the effects of ethyl-eicosapentaenoate in patients with ongoing depression despite apparently adequate treatment with standard drugs. *Arch Gen Psychiatry.* 2002;59(10):913–919.

Peet M, Laugharne JD, Mellor J, Ramchand CN. Essential fatty acid deficiency in erythrocyte membranes from chronic schizophrenic patients, and the clinical effects of dietary supplementation. *Prostaglandins Leukot Essent Fatty Acids.* 1996;55(1–2):71–75.

Peet M, Mellor J. Double-blind placebo controlled trial of n-3 polyunsaturated fatty acids as an adjunct to neuroleptics [abstract]. *Schizophrenia Res.* 1998;29(1–2):160–161.

Petot GJ, Traore F, Debanne SM, et al. Dietary fat intake in mid-adulthood and apolipoprotein E genotype as risk factors for Alzheimer's disease. The 8th International Conference on Alzheimer's Disease and Related Disorders. Stockholm, Sweden. July 20–25, 2002.

Petrek JA, Hudgins LC, Ho M, Bajorunas DR, Hirsch J. Fatty acid composition of adipose tissue, an indication of dietary fatty acids, and breast cancer prognosis. *J Clin Oncol.* 1997;15:1377–1384.

Petrek JA, Hudgins LC, Levine B, Ho M, Hirsch J. Breast cancer risk and fatty acids in breast and abdominal adipose tissue. *J Natl Cancer Inst.* 1994;86:53–56.

Pirmohamed J, James S, Meakin S, et al. Adverse drug reactions as cause of admission to hospital: Prospective analysis of 18,820 patients. *BMJ.* 2004;329(7456):15–19.

Potischman N, Weiss HA, Swanson CA, et al. Diet during adolescence and risk of breast cancer among young women. *J Natl Cancer Inst.* 1998;90:226–233.

Pouliot MC, Després JP, Lemieux S, et al. Waist circumference and abdominal sagittal diameter: Best simple anthropometric indexes of abdominal visceral adipose tissue accumulation and related cardiovascular risk in men and women. *Am J Cardiol.* 1994;73:460–468.

Pouliot MC, Després JP, Nadeau A, et al. Visceral obesity in men: Associations with glucose tolerance, plasma insulin, and lipoprotein levels. *Diabetes.* 1992;41:826–834.

Pratico D, Dogne J-M. Selective cyclooxygenase-2 inhibitors development in cardiovascular medicine. *Circulation.* 2005;112:1073–1079.

Prentice RL. Measurement error and results from analytic epidemiology: Dietary fat and breast cancer. *J Natl Cancer Inst.* 1996;88:1738–1747.

Prentice RL, Sheppard L. Dietary fat and cancer: Consistency of the epidemiologic data, and disease prevention that may follow from a practical reduction in fat consumption. *Cancer Causes Control.* 1990;1:81–97.

Prescott SL. Early origins of allergic disease: A review of processes and influences during early immune development. *Curr Opin Allergy Clin Immunol.* 2003;3(2):125–132.

Priante G, Bordin L, Musacchio E, Clari G, Baggio B. Fatty acids and cytokine mRNA expression in human osteoblastic cells: A specific effect of arachidonic acid. *Clin Sci.* 2002;102:403–409.

Pritchard GA, Jones DL, Mansel RE. Lipids in breast carcinogenesis. *Br J Surg.* 1989; 76:1069–1073.

Pryor M, Slattery ML, Robison LM, Egger M. Adolescent diet and breast cancer in Utah. *Cancer Res.* 1989;49:2161–2167.

Psaty BM, Furberg CD. COX-2 inhibitors: Lessons in drug safety. *N Engl J Med.* 2005;352:1133–1135.

Puri BK, Richardson AJ, Horrobin DF, et al. Eicosapentaenoic acid treatment in schizophrenia associated with symptom remission, normalization of blood fatty acids, reduced neuronal membrane phospholipid turnover and structural brain changes. *Int J Clin Pract.* 2000;54(1):57–63.

Pyorala K. Relationship of glucose tolerance and plasma insulin to the incidence of coronary heart disease: Results from two population studies in Finland. *Diabetes Care.* 1979;2:131–141.

Rambjor GS, Walen AI, Windsor SL, Harris WS. Eicosapentaenoic acid is primarily responsible for the hypotriglyceridemic effect of fish oil in humans. *Lipids.* 1996; 31(suppl):S45–S49.

Raper NR, Cronin JF, Exler J. Omega-3 fatty acid content of the U.S. food supply. *J Am Coll Nutr.* 1992;11:304–308.

Ray WA, Stein CM, Daugherty JR, Hall K, Arbogast PG, Griffin MR. COX-2 selective nonsteroidal anti-inflammatory drugs and risk of serious coronary heart disease. *Lancet.* 2002;360:1071–1073.

Reddy B. Omega-3 fatty acids in colorectal cancer prevention. *Int J Cancer.* 2004; 112(1):1–7.

Reicin AS, Shapiro D, Sperling RS, Barr E, Yu Q. Comparison of cardiovascular thrombotic events in patients with osteoarthritis treated with rofecoxib versus nonselective nonsteroidal antiinflammatory drugs (ibuprofen, diclofenac, and nabumetone). *Am J Cardiol.* 2002;89:204–209.

Richardson AJ, Montgomery P. The Oxford-Durham Study: A randomized controlled trial of dietary supplementation with fatty acids in children with developmental coordination disorder. *Pediatrics.* 2005;115(5):1360–1366.

Richardson AJ, Puri BK. A randomized double-blind, placebo-controlled study of the effects of supplementation with highly unsaturated fatty acids on ADHD-related symptoms in children with specific learning difficulties. *Prog Neuropsychopharmacol Biol Psychiatry.* 2002;26:233–239.

Richardson S, Gerber M, Cenee S. The role of fat, animal protein, and some vitamin consumption in breast cancer: A case control study in southern France. *Int J Cancer.* 1991; 48:1–9.

Rifkind BM, Segal P. Lipid Research Clinics Program reference values for hyperlipidemia and hypolipidemia. *JAMA.* 1983;250:1869–1872.

Rissanen T, Voutilainen S, Nyyssönen K, Lakka TA, Salonen JT. Fish oil–derived fatty acids, docosahexaenoic acid and docosapentaenoic acid, and the risk of acute coronary events: The Kuopio Ischaemic Heart Disease Risk Factor Study. *Circulation.* 2000;102: 2677.

Risk from COX-2 Inhibitors after CABG. *Journal Watch Cardiology.* 2005(401):4.

Rivellese AA, Maffettone A, Iovine C, et al. Long-term effects of fish oil on insulin resistance and plasma lipoproteins in NIDDM patients with hypertriglyceridemia. *Diabetes Care.* 1996;19:1207–1213.

Roberts LJ 2nd, Montine TJ, Markesbery WR, et al. Formation of isoprostane-like compound (neuroprostanes) in vivo from docosahexanoic acid. *J Biol Chem.* 1998;273: 13605.

Robinson E. The health of the James Bay Cree. *Can Fam Physician.* 1988;34:1606–1613.

Roche HM, Gibney MJ. Postprandial triacylglycerolaemia: The effect of low-fat dietary treatment with and without fish oil supplementation. *Eur J Clin Nutr.* 1996;50(9): 617–624.

Rode A, Shephard RJ, Vloshinsky PE, Kuksis A. Plasma fatty acid profiles of Canadian Inuit and Siberian Ganasan. *Arctic Med Res.* 1995;54:10–20.

Rogers AE. Diet and breast cancer: Studies in laboratory animals. *J Nutr.* 1997;127(5; suppl):933S–935S.

Rohan TE, McMichael AJ, Baghurst PA. A population-based case-control study of diet and breast cancer in Australia. *Am J Epidemiol.* 1988;128:478–489.

Ronai Z, Tillotson J, Cohen L. Effect of dietary fatty acids on gene expression in breast cells. *Adv Exp Med Biol.* 1995;375:85–95.

Rose DP. Dietary fatty acids and cancer. *Am J Clin Nutr.* 1997;66(suppl):998S–1003S.

Rose DP. Dietary fatty acids and the prevention of hormone-responsive cancer. *Proc Soc Exp Biol Med.* 1997;216:224–233.

Rose DP. Effects of dietary fatty acids on breast and prostate cancers: Evidence from in vitro experiments and animal studies. *Am J Clin Nutr.* 1997;66(suppl):1513S–1522S.

Rose DP, Boyar AP, Wynder EL. International comparisons of mortality rates for cancer of the breast, ovary, prostate, and colon, and per capita food consumption. *Cancer.* 1986; 58:2363–2371.

Rose DP, Connolly JM. Effects of dietary omega-3 fatty acids on human breast cancer growth and metastases in nude mice. *J Natl Cancer Inst.* 1993;85:1743–1747.

Rose DP, Connolly JM. Omega-3 fatty acids as cancer chemopreventive agents. *Pharmacol Ther.* 1999;83(3):217–244.

Rose DP, Connolly JM, Rayburn J, Coleman M. Influence of diets containing eicosapentaenoic or docosahexaenoic acid on growth and metastasis of breast cancer cells in nude mice. *J Natl Cancer Inst.* 1995;87:587–592.

Rosenson RS, Tangney CC. Antiatherothrombotic properties of statins: Implications for cardiovascular event reduction. *JAMA.* 1998;279:1643–1650.

Ross E. The role of marine fish oils in the treatment of ulcerative colitis. *Nutr Rev.* 1993;51(2):47–49.

Ross JA, Moses AG, Fearon KC. The anti-catabolic effects of n-3 fatty acids. *Curr Opin Clin Nutr Metab Care.* 1999;2:219–226.

Roy I, Meyer F, Gingras L, et al. A double-blind randomized controlled study comparing the efficacy of fish oil and low dose ASA to prevent coronary saphenous vein graft obstruction after CABG [abstract]. *Circulation.* 1991;84:II–285.

Russo J, Gusterson BA, Rogers AE, Russo IH, Wellings SR, van Zwieten MJ. Biology of disease: Comparative study of human and rat mammary tumorigenesis. *Lab Invest.* 1990;62:244–278.

Ryu J, Lerner J, Sullivan J. Unresponsiveness of forearm hemodynamics to omega-3 polyunsaturated fatty acids and aspirin. *Prostaglandins.* 1990;39:339–347.

Sacks FM, Stone PH, Gibson CM, et al. Controlled trial of fish oil for regression of human coronary atherosclerosis. HARP Research Group. *J Am Coll Cardiol.* 1995;25(7): 1492–1498.

Salomon P, Kornbluth AA, Janowitz HD. Treatment of ulcerative colitis with fish oil n-3 omega-fatty acid: An open trial. *J Clin Gastroenterol.* 1990;12(2):157–161.

Salonen JT. Association between cardiovascular death and myocardial infarction and serum selenium in a matched-pair longitudinal study. *Lancet.* 1982;24:175–179.

Salonen JT, Nyyssonen K, Korpela H, Tuomilehto J, Seppanen R, Salonen R. High stored iron levels are associated with excess risk of myocardial infarction in eastern Finnish men. *Circulation.* 1992;86:803–811.

Salonen JT, Seppänen K, Nyyssönen K, et al. Intake of mercury from fish, lipid peroxidation, and the risk of myocardial infarction and coronary, cardiovascular, and any death in eastern Finnish men. *Circulation.* 1995;91:645–655.

Salvi A, Di Stefano O, Sleiman I, et al. Effects of fish oil on serum lipids and lipoprotein(a) levels in heterozygous familial hypercholesterolemia. *Curr Ther Res Clin Exp.* 1993;53(6):717–721.

Salvig JD, Olsen SF, Secher NJ. Effects of fish oil supplementation in late pregnancy on blood pressure: A randomised controlled trial. *BJOG.* 1996;103(6):529–533.

Sanchez-Muniz FJ, Bastida S, Viejo JM, Terpstra AHM. Small supplements of n-3 fatty acids change serum low density lipoprotein composition by decreasing phospholipid and apolipoprotein B concentrations in young adult women. *Eur J Nutr.* 1999;38:20–27.

Sanders TA, Oakley FR, Miller GJ, et al. Influence of n-6 versus n-3 polyunsaturated fatty acids in diets low in saturated fatty acids on plasma lipoproteins and hemostatic factors. *Arterioscler Thromb Vasc Biol.* 1997;17(12):3449–3460.

SanGiovanni JP. Higher intake of omega n-3 long-chain polyunsaturated fatty acid (LCP-UFA) and fish was associated with decreased risk of having neovascular AMD after adjusting for nutrient- and nonnutrient-based predictors and correlates of AMD. Association for Research in Vision and Ophthalmology 2003 annual meeting: Abstract 811/B786, presented May 4, 2003.

Santé Québec. [*Methods*]. In: [*Report of the Santé Québec Health Survey among the Inuit of Nunavik* (*1992*)]. Montréal: Ministère de la Santé et des Services Sociaux du Québec, Gouvernement du Québec, 1994:17–33. [In French.]

Santé Québec. [*Report of the Santé Québec Health Survey among the Inuit of Nunavik* (*1992*): *Diet, a Health Determining Factor.*] Montréal: Ministère de la Santé et des Services Sociaux, Gouvernement du Québec, 1995:47–124. [In French.]

Santé Québec. [*Report on Cardiovascular Health in the Quebec Population, 1990.*] Montréal: Ministère de la Santé et des Services Sociaux, Gouvernement du Québec, 1994. [In French.]

Santos J, Queiros J, Silva F, et al. Effects of fish oil in cyclosporine-treated renal transplant recipients. *Transplant Proc.* 2000;32(8):2605–2608.

Sasaki S, Horacsek M, Kesteloot H. An ecological study of the relationship between dietary fat intake and breast cancer mortality. *Prev Med.* 1993;22:187–202.

Sasaki T, Kobayashi Y, Shimizu J, et al. Effects of dietary n-3-to-n-6 polyunsaturated fatty acid ratio on mammary carcinogenesis in rats. *Nutr Cancer.* 1998;30:137–143.

Schaefer EJ, Lamon-Fava S, Spiegelman D, et al. Changes in plasma lipoprotein concentration and composition in response to a low-fat, high-fiber diet are associated with changes in serum estrogen concentrations in premenopausal women. *Metabolism.* 1995;44:749–756.

Schaefer EJ, Lichtenstein AH, Lamon-Fava S, et al. Effects of National Education Program Step 2 diets relatively high or relatively low in fish-derived fatty acids on plasma lipoproteins in middle-aged and elderly subjects. *Am J Clin Nutr.* 1996;63:234–241.

Schlanger S, Shinitzky M, Yam D. Diet enriched with omega-3 fatty acids alleviates convulsion symptoms in epilepsy patients. *Epilepsia.* 2002;43(1):103–104.

Schmidt EB, Skou HA, Christensen JH, Dyerberg J. N-3 fatty acids from fish and coronary artery disease: Implications for public health. *Public Health Nutr.* 2000;3:91–98.

Schmidt EB, Varming K, Ernst E, Madsen P, Dyerberg J. Dose-response studies on the effect of n-3 polyunsaturated fatty acids on lipids and haemostasis. *Thromb Haemost.* February 19, 1990;63(1):1–5.

Schmidt R. Early inflammation and dementia: A 25-year follow-up of the Honolulu-Asia Aging Study. *Ann Neurol.* 2002;52(2):168–174.

Schnitzer TJ, Burmester GR, Mysler E, et al. Comparison of lumiracoxib with naproxen and ibuprofen in the Therapeutic Arthritis Research and Gastrointestinal Event Trial (TARGET), reduction in ulcer complications: Randomised controlled trial. *Lancet.* 2004; 364:665–674.

Schraer C, Adler A, Mayer A, Halderson K, Trimble B. Diabetes complications and mortality among Alaska natives: 8 years of observation. *Diabetes Care.* 1997;20:314–21.

Schulze MB, Rimm EB, Li T, Rifai N, Stampfer MJ, Hu FB. C-reactive protein and incident cardiovascular events among men with diabetes. *Diabetes Care.* 2004;27:889–894.

Sears B. *The Zone.* New York: HarperCollins; 1995.

Seddon JM, Cote J, Rosner B. Progression of age-related macular degeneration: Association with dietary fat, transunsaturated fat, nuts, and fish intake. *Arch Ophthalmol.* 2003; 121(12):1728–1737.

Sellmayer A, Witzgall H, Lorenz RL, et al. Effects of dietary fish oil on ventricular premature complexes. *Am J Cardiol.* 1995;76(12):974–977.

Serhan CN, Clish CB, Brannon J, Colgan SP, Chiang N, Gronert K. Novel functional sets of lipid-derived mediators with antiinflammatory actions generated from omega-3 fatty acids via cyclooxygenase 2-nonsteroidal antiinflammatory drugs and transcellular processing. *J Exp Med.* 2000;192:1197–1204.

Serhan CN, Jain A, Marleau S, Clish C, Kantarci A, Behbehani B, Colgan SP, Stahl GL, Merched A, Petasis NA, Chan L, Van Dyke TE. Reduced inflammation and tissue damage in transgenic rabbits overexpressing 15-lipoxygenase and endogenous anti-inflammatory lipid mediators. *J. Immunol.* 2003;171:6856–6865.

Shaya FT, Blume SW, Blanchette CM, Mullins CD, Weir MR. Cardiovascular risk of selective cyclooxygenase-2 inhibitors compared to other nonsteroidal anti-inflammatory agents: An observational study of a Medicaid population. *Pharmacoepidemiol Drug Saf.* 2004;13:S234–S234.

Shekelle RB, Missel L, Paul O, Shryock AM, Stamler L. Fish consumption and mortality from coronary heart disease. *N Engl J Med.* 1985;313:820.

Shoda R, Matsueda K, Yamato S, Umeda N. Epidemiologic analysis of Crohn disease in Japan: Increased dietary intake of *n*-6 polyunsaturated fatty acids and animal protein relates to the increased incidence of Crohn disease in Japan. *Am J Clin Nutr.* 1996;63:741–745.

Shultz TD. Physiological free fatty acid concentrations do not increase free estradiol in plasma. *J Clin Endocrinol Metab.* 1991;72:65–68.

Shun-Zhang Y, Rui-Fang L, Da-Dao X, Howe GR. A case-control study of dietary and nondietary risk factors for breast cancer in Shanghai. *Cancer Res.* 1990;50:5017–5021.

Simard A, Vobecky J, Vobecky JS. Nutrition and lifestyle factors in fibrocystic disease and cancer of the breast. *Cancer Detect Prev.* 1990;14:567–572.

Simon J, Hodgkins M, Browner W, Neuhaus J, Bernert J, Hulley S. Serum fatty acids and the risk of coronary heart disease. *Am J Epidemiol.* 1995;142:469–476.

Simon JA, Fong J, Bernert JT Jr, et al. Serum fatty acids and the risk of stroke. *Stroke.* 1995;26(5):778–782.

Simonsen N, van't Veer P, Strain JJ, et al. Adipose tissue omega-3 and omega-6 fatty acid content and breast cancer in the EURAMIC Study. *Am J Epidemiol.* 1998;147:342–352.

Simonsen NR, Fernandez-Crehuet Navajas J, Martin-Moreno JM, et al. Tissue stores of individual monounsaturated fatty acids and breast cancer: The EURAMIC Study. *Am J Clin Nutr.* 1998;68:134–141.

Simopoulos AP. Evolutionary aspects of diet, essential fatty acids and cardiovascular disease. *Eur Heart J.* 2001; 3(suppl D):D8–D21.

Sinclair AJ, Murphy KJ, Li D. Marine lipids: Overview "news insights and lipid composition of Lyprinol." *Allerg Immunol* (Paris). September 2000;32(7):261–271.

Singer P, Melzer S, Goschel M, et al. Fish oil amplifies the effect of propranolol in mild essential hypertension. *Hypertension.* 1990;16(6):682–691.

Singh RB, Niaz MA, Sharma JP, Kumar R, Rastogi V, Moshiri M. Randomized, double-blind, placebo-controlled trial of fish oil and mustard oil in patients with suspected acute myocardial infarction: The Indian experiment of infarct survival–4. *Cardiovasc Drugs Ther.* 1997;11(3):485–491.

Siscovick DS, Raghunathan TE, King I, et al. Dietary intake and cell membrane levels of long-chain n-3 polyunsaturated fatty acids and the risk of primary cardiac arrest. *JAMA.* 1995;274:1363–1367.

Skoldstam L, Borjesson O, Kjallman A, et al. Effect of six months of fish oil supplementation in stable rheumatoid arthritis: A double-blind, controlled study. *Scand J Rheumatol.* 1992;21(4):178–185.

Smith LL, van Lier JE. Sterol metabolism, IX: 26-hydroxycholesterol levels in the human aorta. *Atherosclerosis.* 1970;12:1–14.

Smuts CM, Huang M, Mundy D, Plasse T, Major S, Carlson SE. A randomized trial of docosahexaenoic acid supplementation during the third trimester of pregnancy. *Obstet Gynecol.* 2003;101(3):469–479.

Solomon SD, McMurray JJV, Pfeffer MA, et al. Cardiovascular risk associated with celecoxib in a clinical trial for colorectal adenoma prevention. *N Engl J Med.* 2005;352(11): 1071-1080.

Soyland E, Funk J, Rajka G, et al. Dietary supplementation with very long-chain n-3 fatty acids in patients with atopic dermatitis: A double-blind, multicentre study. *Br J Dermatol.* 1994;130(6):757-764.

Soyland E, Funk J, Rajka G, et al. Effect of dietary supplementation with very-long-chain n-3 fatty acids in patients with psoriasis. *N Engl J Med.* 1993;328:1812-1816.

Sperling RI, Weinblatt M, Robin JL, et al. Effects of dietary supplementation with marine fish oil on leukocyte lipid mediator generation and function in rheumatoid arthritis. *Arthritis Rheum.* 1987;30(9):988-997.

Stacpoole PW, Alig J, Ammon L, et al. Dose-response effects of dietary fish oil on carbohydrate and lipid metabolism in hypertriglyceridemia [abstract]. *Diabetes.* 1988;37(suppl 1):12A.

Stacpoole PW, Alig J, Ammon L, et al. Dose-response effects of dietary marine oil on carbohydrate and lipid metabolism in normal subjects and patients with hypertriglyceridemia. *Metabolism.* 1989;38(10):946-956.

Staessen L, De Henauw S, De Bacquer D, De Backer G, Van Peteghem C. Consumption of fatty acids in Belgium and its relationship with cancer mortality. *Cancer Lett.* 1997; 114:109-111.

Stenius-Aarniala B, Aro A, Hakulinen A, et al. Evening primrose oil and fish oil are ineffective as supplementary treatment of bronchial asthma. *Ann Allergy.* 1989;62(6): 534-537.

Stenson WF, Cort D, Beeken W, et al. A trial of fish oil supplemented diet in ulcerative colitis [abstract]. *Gastroenterology.* 1990;98(suppl):A475.

Stenson WF, Cort D, Rodgers J, et al. Dietary supplementation with fish oil in ulcerative colitis. *Ann Intern Med.* 1992;116(8):609-614.

Stevens L, Zhang W, Peck L, et al. EFA Supplementation in children with inattention, hyperactivity, and other disruptive behaviours. *Lipids.* 2003;38:1007-1021.

Stevens LJ, Zentall SS, Deck JL, et al. Essential fatty-acid metabolism in boys with attention-deficit hyperactivity disorder. *Am J Clin Nutr.* 1995;62:761-768.

Stewart WF, Kawas C, Corrada M, Metter EJ. Risk of Alzheimer's disease and duration of NSAID use. *Neurology.* 1997;48(3):626-632.

Stoll AL, Severus WE, Freeman MP, et al. Omega 3 fatty acids in bipolar disorder: A preliminary double-blind, placebo-controlled trial. *Arch Gen Psychiatry.* 1999;56(5):407-412.

Stone NJ. Fish consumption, fish oil, lipids, and coronary heart disease. *Circulation.* 1996;94(9):2337-2340.

Stoof TJ, Korstanje MJ, Bilo HJ, et al. Does fish oil protect renal function in cyclosporin-treated psoriasis patients? *J Intern Med.* 1989;226(6):437-441.

Storlien LH, Kriketos AD, Calvert GD, Baur LA, Jenkins AB. Fatty acids, triglycerides and syndromes of insulin resistance. *Prostaglandins Leukot Essent Fatty Acids.* 1997;57:3 79-385.

Strong AM, Hamill E. The effect of combined fish oil and evening primrose oil (Efamol Marine) on the remission phase of psoriasis: A 7-month double-blind randomized placebo-controlled trial. *J Derm Treatment*. 1993;4:33–36.

Studer M, Briel M, Leimenstoll B, et al. Effect of different antilipidemic agents and diets on mortality. *Arch Intern Med*. 2005;165:725–730.

Su KP, Huang SY, Chiu CC, et al. Omega-3 fatty acids in major depressive disorder. A preliminary double-blind, placebo-controlled trial. *Eur Neuropsychopharmacol*. 2003; 13(4):267–271.

Suadicani P, Hein HO, Gyntelberg F. Serum selenium concentration and risk of ischaemic heart disease in a prospective cohort study of 3,000 males. *Atherosclerosis*. 1992;96: 33–42.

Suzukawa M, Abbey M, Howe PR, Nestel PJ. Effects of fish oil fatty acids on low density lipoprotein size, oxidizability, and uptake by macrophages. *J Lipid Res*. 1995;3: 473–484.

Swank RL, Lerstad O, Strom A, Backer J. Multiple sclerosis in rural Norway: Its geographic and occupational incidence in relation to nutrition. *N Engl J Med*. 1952;246(19): 722–728.

Sweny P, Wheeler DC, Lui SF, et al. Dietary fish oil supplements preserve renal function in renal transplant recipients with chronic vascular rejection. *Nephrol Dial Transplant*. 1989;4(12):1070–1075.

Takata T, Minoura T, Takada H, et al. Specific inhibitory effect of dietary eicosapentaenoic acid on N-nitroso-N-methylurea-induced mammary carcinogenesis in female Sprague-Dawley rats. *Carcinogenesis*. 1990;11;2015–2019.

Tanskanen A, Hibbeln JR, Hintikka J, et al. Fish consumption, depression, and suicidality in a general population. *Arch Gen Psychiatry*. 2001;58(5):512–513.

Tar L, Tar K. Stop prescribing cox-2 inhibitors? A medico-legal analysis. *Allegheny Cty Med Soc Bull*. June 2005:293–296.

Tato F, Keller C, Wolfram G. Effects of fish oil concentrate on lipoproteins and apolipoproteins in familial combined hyperlipidemia. *Clin Investig*. 1993;71(4):314–318.

Telang NT, Inoue S, Bradlow HL, Osborne MP. Negative growth regulation of oncogene-transformed mammary epithelial cells by tumor inhibitors. *Adv Exp Med Biol*. 1997;400A:409–418.

Tenkanen L, Pietila K, Manninen V, Mantarri M. The triglyceride issue revisited: Findings from the Helsinki Heart Study. *Arch Intern Med*. 1994;154:2714–2720.

Terry P, Lichtenstein P, Feychting M, Ahlbom A, Wolk A. Fatty fish consumption and risk of prostate cancer. *Lancet*. 2001;357(9270):1764–1766.

Thien FC, Mencia-Huerta JM, Lee TH. Dietary fish oil effects on seasonal hay fever and asthma in pollen- sensitive subjects. *Am Rev Respir Dis*. 1993;147(5):1138–1143.

Thies F, Garry JM, Yaqoob P, et al. Association of n-3 polyunsaturated fatty acids with stability of atherosclerotic plaques: A randomized controlled trial. *Lancet*. 2003;361: 477–485.

Thorngren M, Gustafson A. Effects of 11-week increases in dietary eicosapentaenoic acid on bleeding time, lipids and platelet aggregation. *Lancet.* 1981;2(8257):1190–1193.

Tisdale MJ. Wasting in cancer. *J Nutr.* January 1999;129(1S; suppl):243S–246S.

Toniolo P, Riboli E, Protta F, Charrel M, Cappa APM. Calorie-providing nutrients and risk of breast cancer. *J Natl Cancer Inst.* 1989;81:278–286.

Toniolo P, Riboli E, Shore RE, Pasternack BS. Consumption of meat, animal products, protein and fat and risk of breast cancer: A prospective study in New York. *Epidemiology.* 1994;5:391–397.

Topol EJ. Failing the public health: Rofecoxib, Merck, and the FDA. *N Engl J Med.* 2004;351:1707–1709.

Trichopoulou A, Katsouyanni K, Stuver S, et al. Consumption of olive oil and specific food groups in relation to breast cancer risk in Greece. *J Natl Cancer Inst.* 1995; 87:110–116.

Trivedi KA, Dana MR, Gilbard JP, Buring JE, Schaumberg DA. Dietary omega-3 fatty acid intake and risk of clinically diagnosed dry eye syndrome in women [abstract]. *Invest Ophthalmol Vis Sci.* 2003;44:811.

Tsubura A, Uehara N, Kiyozuka Y, Shikata N. Dietary factors modifying breast cancer risk and relation to time of intake. *J Mammary Gland Biol Neoplasia.* 2005;10(1):87–100.

Tsuda H, Iwahori Y, Asamoto M, et al. Demonstration of organotropic effects of chemo-preventive agents in multiorgan carcinogenesis models. *IARC Sci Publ.* 1996;139: 143–150.

Tulleken JE, Limburg PC, Muskiet FA, et al. Vitamin E status during dietary fish oil sup-plementation in rheumatoid arthritis. *Arthritis Rheum.* 1990;33(9):1416–1419.

Ullmann D, Connor WE, Illingworth DR, et al. Additive effects of lovastatin and fish oil in familial hypercholesterolemia [abstract]. *Arteriosclerosis.* 1990;10(5):846a.

U.S. Department of Agriculture Nutrient Data Laboratory [database online]. Available at: www.nalusda.gov/fnic/foodcomp. Accessed online March 29, 2004.

U.S. Department of Health, Education, and Welfare. *Lipid and Lipoprotein Analysis: Manual of Laboratory Operation.* Lipid Research Clinics Program. Washington, DC: USD-HEW, 1982.

U.S. Food and Drug Administration. *What You Need to Know about Mercury in Fish and Shellfish.* FDA/CFSAN Consumer Advisory (EPA-823-R-04-005). March 2004. Available at: www.cfsan.fda.gov/ ~ dms/admehg3.html.

U.S. Food and Drug Administration Center for Food Safety and Applied Nutrition. *Agency Response Letter GRAS Notice No. GRN 000105.* October 15, 2002. Available at: www.cfsan.fda.gov/ ~ rdb/opa-g105.html.

U.S. Food and Drug Administration Center for Food Safety and Applied Nutrition. *Letter Regarding Dietary Supplement Health Claim for Omega-3 Fatty Acids and Coronary Heart Disease.* October 31, 2000. Available at: www.cfsan.fda.gov/ ~ dms/ds-ltr11.html.

U.S. Food and Drug Administration Center for Food Safety and Applied Nutrition. *Letter Responding to Health Claim Petition Dated November 3, 2003 (Martek Petition): Omega-*

3 Fatty Acids and Reduced Risk of Coronary Heart Disease (docket no. 2003Q-0401). September 8, 2004. Available at: www.cfsan.fda.gov/~dms/ds-ltr37.html.

Vancheri C, Mastruzzo C, Sortino MA, Crimi N. The lung as a privileged site for the beneficial actions of PGE_2. *Trends Immunol.* 2004;25:40–46.

van den Brandt PA, van't Veer P, Goldbohm RA, et al. A prospective cohort study on dietary fat and the risk of postmenopausal breast cancer. *Cancer Res.* 1993;53:75–82.

van der Tempel H, Tulleken JE, Limburg PC, et al. Effects of fish oil supplementation in rheumatoid arthritis. *Ann Rheum Dis.* 1990;49(2):76–80.

van der Heide JJ, Bilo HJ, Donker JM, et al. Effect of dietary fish oil on renal function and rejection in cyclosporine-treated recipients of renal transplants. *N Engl J Med.* 1993;329(11):769–773.

Vargova V, Vesely R, Sasinka M, Torok C. [Will administration of omega-3 unsaturated fatty acids reduce the use of nonsteroidal antirheumatic agents in children with chronic juvenile arthritis?] *Cas Lek Cesk.* 1998;137:651–653. [Article in Slovak.]

Vatten LJ, Sollvoll K, Loken EB. Frequency of meat and fish intake and risk of breast cancer in a prospective study of 14,500 Norwegian women. *Int J Cancer.* 1990;46:12–15.

Ventura HO, Milani RV, Lavie CJ, et al. Cyclosporine-induced hypertension: efficacy of omega-3 fatty acids in patients after cardiac transplantation. *Circulation.* 1993;88(5, part 2):II_281–II_285.

Voigt RG, Llorente AM, Beretta MC, et al. Docosahexaenoic acid (DHA) supplementation does not improve the symptoms of attention-deficit/hyperactivity disorder (ADHD). *Pediatr Res.* 1999;45:17A.

Volker D, Fitzgerald P, Major G, Garg M. Efficacy of fish oil concentrate in the treatment of rheumatoid arthritis. *J Rheumatol.* 2000;27:2343–2346.

von Schacky C, Angerer P, Kothny W, Theisen K, Mudra H. The effect of dietary omega-3 fatty acids on coronary atherosclerosis: a randomized, double-blind, placebo-controlled trial. *Ann Intern Med.* 1999;130:554–562.

Walton AJ, Snaith ML, Locniskar M, Cumberland AG, Morrow WJ, Isenberg DA. Dietary fish oil and the severity of symptoms in patients with systemic lupus erythematosus. *Ann Rheum Dis.* 1991;50(7):463–466.

Wang C, Chung M, Lichtenstein A, et al. *Omega-3 Fatty Acids Effects on Cardiovascular Disease* [summary]. Evidence Report/Technology Assessment no. 94 (AHRQ 04-E009-1). Rockville, MD: Agency for Healthcare Research and Quality; 2004.

Wein E, Freeman MMR, Makus JC. Use and preference for traditional foods among the Belcher Island Inuit. *Arctic.* 1996;49:256–264.

Weksler BB. Omega 3 fatty acids have multiple antithrombotic effects. *World Rev Nutr Diet.* 1994;76:47–50.

Welsch CW. Interrelationship between dietary lipids and calories and experimental mammary gland tumorigenesis. *Cancer.* 1994;74:1055–1062.

Welty TK, Lee ET, Yeh J, et al. Cardiovascular disease risk factors among American Indians: The Strong Heart Study. *Am J Epidemiol.* 1995;142:269–287.

White PF. Changing role of COX-2 inhibitors in the perioperative period: Is parecoxib really the answer? *Anesth Analg.* 2005;100:1306–1308.

Wigmore SJ, Barber MD, Ross JA et al. Effect of oral eicosapentaenoic acid on weight loss in patients with pancreatic cancer. *Nutr Cancer.* 2000;36:177–184.

Wigmore SJ, Ross JA, Falconer JS, et al. The effect of polyunsaturated fatty acids on the progress of cachexia in patients with pancreatic cancer. *Nutrition.* January 1996;12(1; suppl):S27–S30.

Willett W. Food frequency methods. In: Willett W, ed. *Nutritional Epidemiology.* 2nd ed. New York: Oxford University Press; 1998:74–100.

Willett W. Response to Wynder et al.'s paper on dietary fat and breast cancer. *J Clin Epidemiol.* 1994;47:223–226.

Willett W. Specific fatty acids and risks of breast and prostate cancer: Dietary intake. *Am J Clin Nutr.* 1997;66(suppl):1557S–1563S.

Willett WC. Dietary fat intake and cancer risk: A controversial and instructive story. *Semin Cancer Biolo.* 1998;8:245–253.

Willett WC, Ascherio A. Trans fatty acids: Are the effects only marginal? *Am J Public Health.* 1994;84:722–724.

Willett WC, Hunter DJ, Stampfer MJ, et al. Dietary fat and fiber in relation to risk of breast cancer. *JAMA.* 1992;268:2037–2044.

Willett WC, Stampfer MJ, Colditz GA, Rosner BA, Hennekens CH, Speizer FE. Dietary fat and the risk of breast cancer. *New Engl J Med.* 1987;316:22–28.

Willett WC, Stampfer MJ, Manson JE, et al. Intake of trans fatty acids and risk of coronary heart disease among women. *Lancet.* 1993;341:581–585.

Williams MA, Zingheim RW, King IB, Zebelman AM. Omega-3 fatty acids in maternal erythrocytes and risk of preeclampsia. *Epidemiology.* May 1995;6(3):232–237.

Wilson PW. An epidemiologic perspective of systemic hypertension, ischemic heart disease, and heart failure. *Am J Cardiol.* 1997;80:3J–8J.

Wolk A, Bergstrom R, Hunter D, et al. A prospective study of association of monounsaturated fat and other types of fat with risk of breast cancer. *Arch Intern Med.* 1998; 158:41–45.

Woodman RJ, Mori TA, Burke V, Puddey IB, Watts GF, Beilin LJ. Effects of purified eicosapentaenoic and docosahexaenoic acids on glycemic control, blood pressure, and serum lipids in type 2 diabetic patients with treated hypertension. *Am J Clin Nutr.* 2002; 76:1007–1015.

Woods RK, Raven JM, Walters EH, Abramson MJ, Thien FC. Fatty acid levels and risk of asthma in young adults. *Thorax.* 2004;59(2):105–110.

Woods RK, Thien FC, Abramson MJ. Dietary marine fatty acids (fish oil) for asthma in adults and children. *Cochrane Database Syst Rev.* 2002;(3):CD001283.

Wooten GF, Currie LJ, Bovbjerg VE, Lee JK, Patrie J. Are men at greater risk for Parkinson's disease than women? *J Neurol Neurosurg Psychiatry.* 2004;75:637–639.

World Cancer Research Fund and the American Institute for Cancer Research. *Food, Nutrition and the Prevention of Cancer: A Global Perspective.* Washington, DC: American Institute for Cancer Research; 1997; 252–287.

World Health Organization. *International Classification of Diseases.* 9th rev. Geneva: WHO, 1977.

Wynder EL, Cohen LA, Muscat JE, Winters B, Dwyer JT, Blackburn G. Breast cancer: Weighing the evidence for a promoting role of dietary fat. *J Natl Cancer Inst.* 1997; 89:766–775.

Wynder EL, Cohen LA, Rose DP, Stellman SD. Dietary fat and breast cancer: Where do we stand on the evidence? *J Clin Epidemiol.* 1994;47:217–222.

Wynder EL, Cohen LA, Rose DP, Stellman SD. Response to Dr. Walter Willett's dissent. *J Clin Epidemiol.* 1994;47:227–230.

Yam D, Bott-Kanner G, Genin I, Shinitzky M, Klainman E. [The effect of omega-3 fatty acids on risk factors for cardiovascular diseases.] *Harefuah.* 2001;140(12):1156–1158, 1230. [Article in Hebrew.]

Yamada T, Strong JP, Ishii T, et al. Atherosclerosis and omega-3 fatty acids in the populations of a fishing village and a farming village in Japan. *Atherosclerosis.* 2000;153(2): 469–481.

Yamori Y, Nara Y, Iritani N, Workman RJ, Inagami T. Comparison of serum phospholipid fatty acids among fishing and farming Japanese populations and American islanders. *J Nutr Sci Vitaminol* (Tokyo). 1985;31:417–422.

Yang LY, Kuksis A, Myher JJ. Lipolysis of menhaden oil triacylglycerols and the corresponding fatty acid alkyl esters by pancreatic lipase in vitro: A reexamination. *J Lipid Res.* 1990;31(1):137–147.

Yarnell JWG, Sweetnam PM, Marks V, Teale JD, Bolton CH. Insulin in ischaemic heart disease: Are associations explained by triglyceride concentrations? The Caerphilly Prospective Study. *Br Heart J.* 1994;71:293–296.

Young GS, Maharaj NJ, Conquer JA. Blood phospholipid fatty acid analysis of adults with and without attention deficit/hyperactivity disorder. *Lipids.* 2004;39(2):117–123.

Young TK, Gerrard JM, O'Neil JD. Plasma phospholipid fatty acids in the central Canadian Arctic: Biocultural explanations for ethnic differences. *Am J Phys Anthropol.* 1999; 109:9–18.

Yuan J-M, Wang Q-S, Ross RK, Henderson BE, Yu MC. Diet and breast cancer in Shanghai and Tianjin, China. *Br J Cancer.* 1995;71:1353–1358.

Zanarini MC, Frankenburg FR. Omega-3 fatty acid treatment of women with borderline personality disorder: A double-blind, placebo-controlled pilot study. *Am J Psychiatry.* 2003;160(1):167–169.

Zaridze D, Lifanova Y, Maximovitch D, Day NE, Duffy SW. Diet, alcohol consumption and reproductive factors in a case-control study of breast cancer in Moscow. *Int J Cancer.* 1991;48:493–501.

Zhang J, Sasaki S, Amano K, et al. Fish consumption and mortality from all causes, ischemic heart disease, and stroke: An ecological study. *Prev Med.* 1999;28(5):520–529.

Zhang S, Folsom AR, Sellers TA, Kushi LH, Potter JD. Better breast cancer survival for postmenopausal women who are less overweight and eat less fat. *Cancer.* 1995;76: 275–283.

Zhu ZR, Agren J, Mannisto S, Pietinen P, Eskelinen M, Syrjanen K, Uusitupa M. Fatty acid composition of breast adipose tissue in breast cancer patients and in patients with benign breast disease. *Nutr Cancer.* 1995;24:151–160.

Index

Acetaminophen, 98
Adenoma Prevention with
    Celecoxib (APC), 29
Adipokines, 68
Adverse Drug Reactions
    (ADRs), 20
Advil. *See* Ibuprofen.
Agency for Healthcare
    Research and Quality
    (AHRQ), 72
AHRQ Report. *See Effects of
    Omega-3 Fatty Acids on
    Cardiovascular Risk
    Factors and Intermediate
    Markers of Cardiovascular
    Disease.*
Alcohol, 22
Aleve, 14
Algae, 41, 50
Allergies, 22, 86, 116, 117
Alpha-linolenic acid, 35, 38,
    41, 50, 76
Alzheimer, Alois, 96
Alzheimer's disease, 96–99
American Heart Association
    (AHA), 49, 76
Anisidine value (AV), 112
Anti-inflammatories, 1–4, 14,
    33
Antioxidants, 111
Apolipoprotein B, 75
Apolipoprotein E (apoE), 98
APPROVe (Adenomatous
    Polyp Prevention on
    Vioxx), 28–29
Arachidonic acid (AA), 11, 14,
    16, 40, 43–44, 46–47, 113

Arrhythmias, 65, 71, 73, 75,
    76
Arteries, 22, 69, 71–72
Arthritis, 27, 29
    osteo, 82–83
    rheumatoid, 80–82, 115
Arugula, 50
Ascorbyl palmitate, 112
Asperger's syndrome, 95
Aspirin, 15, 19, 21–23, 32,
    47, 98, 119
    complications from, 22–23
Asthma, 14, 22, 86–88
Atherosclerosis, 110, 111
Attention-deficit hyperactivity
    disorder (ADHD), 93–94
Autism, 95, 96
Autoimmune diseases, 79,
    80, 84–86, 89

Bang, H. O., 58, 61
Bayer Pharmaceutical
    Company, 21
Beta-amyloid, 96, 98
Bextra, 2, 24, 29, 30
Bile acid, 105
Bipolar disorder, 101
Blood, 70–71, 72, 117–118
    clots and clotting, 10, 22,
    29–31, 72, 76, 117, 118–119
    pressure, 72, 73, 76, 115, 119
    vessels, 69, 70, 86
Bone marrow, 8
Bucher, H. C., 64, 74

C-reactive protein (CRP), 8,
    74, 77–78, 98, 104

Cachexia, 105
Cancer, 102–105, 111
    breast, 103–104
    colorectal, 104–105
    prostate, 102–103
Cardiovascular disease, 21–22,
    27–28, 29, 30–31, 37, 48,
    50, 58, 60–68, 78–79
    clinical studies, 60–64
Celebrex, 2, 23, 24, 29, 30
Celecoxib. *See* Celebrex.
Cells, 6, 8, 38–40
    aggregated, 16
    brain, 77
    endothelial, 71
    red blood, 16
    See also Eicosanoids;
    Leukocytes.
Center for Drug Evaluation
    and Research (CDER), 19
Chemotaxis, 12
Chemotherapy, 105–106
Cheuvront, Samuel, 46
Children and infants, 54, 86,
    91, 116–117
Cholesterol, 37, 43, 49,
    68–69, 74–75, 111
    high-density lipoproteins
    (HDL), 69
    low-level lipoproteins
    (LDL), 66, 68–69
    very-low-density
    lipoproteins (vLDL),
    68–69, 79
Clopidogrel (Plavix), 119
Colitis, ulcerative, 83, 84
Complement system, 7, 8

Coronary artery bypass
  grafting (CABG), 29,
  64–65
Coronary artery disease
  (CAD), 67, 114
Coronary heart disease (CHD).
  See Cardiovascular
  disease.
Corticosteroids, 20
COX. *See* Cyclooxygenase
  (COX).
COX-2 inhibitors, 2, 23,
  24–32
Crohn's disease, 83, 84
Cyclooxygenase (COX), 1,
  11, 12, 15, 21, 23–26,
  43–44, 47
Cyclosporine nephrotoxicity,
  115–116
Cysteine proteases, 70
Cytokines, 15, 47, 70

D-series resolvins, 47
Dental hygiene, 70
Depression, 99–101
  postpartum, 92, 101
Dermatitis, atopic, 90
Developmental coordination
  disorder (DCD), 95
DHA. *See* Docosahaenoic
  acid (DHA).
Diabetes, 69, 73, 78–80
Diet, 1, 14–15, 16, 36–37, 40,
  41, 42, 48–49, 58, 61, 68,
  85–86, 92, 93, 97, 98–99,
  102–103, 105
  Mediterranean, 61
  Zone, 46
Dietary supplements, health
  claims, 56–57
Docosahexaenoic acid (DHA),
  11, 41, 43–44, 47, 49, 50,
  75, 77, 91, 92, 97, 98,
  100, 108
  dosages, 55, 116
Dopamine, 99
Drugs, pharmaceutical, 18–32
Dry eye syndrome, 88–89
Dyerberg, J., 58, 61

E-series resolvins, 47
Eczema, 90

*Effects of Omega-3 Fatty Acids
  on Cardiovascular Risk
  Factors and Intermediate
  Markers of Cardiovascular
  Disease,* 72–75
Eicosanoids, 8–15, 34, 40, 45
Eicosapentaenoic acid (EPA),
  11, 41, 43–44, 47, 49, 50,
  75, 108, 113
  dosages, 55, 115
EPA. *See* Eicosapentaenoic
  acid (EPA).
Essential fatty acids (EFAs),
  10–12, 33–47, 55, 61
  monounsaturated, 35, 103
  polyunsaturated, 35, 38,
  111
  saturated, 35, 49, 99, 103
  unsaturated, 35, 36
  See also Omega-3 fatty
  acids; Omega-6 fatty
  acids.
Ethyl esters, 109–110
Exercise, 75

Fats, trans, 36–38, 48, 49
Fatty acids. *See* Essential fatty
  acids (EFAs).
Fever, 13, 15
Fibrinogen, 74
Fibroblasts, 46
Fish, 42, 49, 50–54, 78–79,
  87–88, 89–90, 91–92, 100,
  113
  farmed, 51
Fish oil, 2, 41, 50, 54–56, 60,
  118
  dosages, 113–117
  oxidation, 110–113
  potency, 108–110
  purity, 107–108
  side effects and
  contraindications,
  117–119
  storage, 112
Flaxseeds, 14, 76
Food Guide Pyramid, 49
Free radicals, 71, 110

Gastic mucosa, 24
Gastrointestinal complications,
  20, 22, 23, 24–26, 119

Genes, 47
Glucose, 69, 73
Gluten, 86
Graham, John D., 48–49

Hearing, 22
Heart attacks, 21–22, 27–29,
  58, 61, 81
Heart disease. *See*
  Cardiovascular disease.
Heparin, 119
Hippocrates, 21
Histamines, 6–7
Hydrocarbons, 34
Hydrogenation, 35–36, 37
Hydroperoxides, 110, 110
Hypertriglyceridemia, 66–67,
  114

Ibuprofen, 14, 27
Immune system, 5, 67, 69
Immunoglobulin E (IgE), 87
Inflammation, 1, 2–3, 6–17,
  20, 43, 46, 67–68, 70, 71,
  73, 77–78, 80, 97
  chronic, 16–17, 18, 33, 43,
  45
  classic, 6–15
  signs of , 6
  systematic, 15–16
Inflammatory bowel disease,
  83–84
Interleukin-1 (IL-1), 15–16
International normalized ratio
  (INR), 118
Intima, 69–70
Inuit effect, 70
Inuit Eskimos, 58, 118

Joints, 29
  cartilage, 82, 83

Kinins, 7

Lands, W. E. M., 46
Lecithin, 112
Leukocytes, 8
Leukotrienes (LT), 9, 11, 14,
  34, 43, 87
Lifestyle, 1, 68, 102
Linoleic acid, 35, 36, 38, 40,
  41

Lipid oxidation, 110–113
Lipids, 69, 70
Lipoproteins, 68–70
Lipoxygenase (LOX), 11, 14, 43–44

Macrophages, 16, 17, 46, 69–70
Macular degeneration, 89–90
Maroon, Joseph, 2
Matrix metalloproteinases, 70, 81–82
Medicine
  anti-aging 60
  complementary, 59
  preventive, 60
  traditional, 59
Mercury, 51, 54, 92
Milk and dairy products, 86
Molecular distillation, 107–108
Motrin. *See* Ibuprofen.
Multiple sclerosis (MS), 85–86

Naproxen, 24, 27
Neutrophils, 16
NFαB, 47
Nonsteroid anti-inflammatories (NSAIDs), 1–2, 12, 20, 21, 22, 23–32, 81
  side effects, 23, 24–25
  See also Aspirin.

Obesity, 68, 78
Oils, 42, 50, 100, 112–113
  canola, 76, 112
  cod liver, 110, 119
  corn, 35
  hydrogenated, 37
  safflower, 112
  See also Fish oil.
Oleic acid, 103
Omega-3 fatty acids, 3, 10–12, 14, 38, 40, 41, 43, 47, 48, 49, 55, 75
Omega-3 index, 113–114
Omega-6 fatty acids, 10–12, 14, 38, 40–41, 43, 44, 81
Oxidative stress, 96, 97

Pain, 6, 10, 12, 20, 23, 24, 27, 82
  back, 29
  menstrual, 92–93
  spine, 82
Parkinson's disease, 99
Percutaneous transluminal coronary angioplasty (PTCA), 65
Peroxide value (PV), 112
Peroxides. *See* Hydroperoxides.
Phagocytes, 12
Phagocytosis, 12
Phospholipids, 10, 43, 91, 102
Plaques, 69–70, 72, 74, 76, 110
Platelets, 21, 69, 70,71
Polychlorinated biphenyls (PCBs), 51
Polyps, 28, 29
Pregnancy, 54, 91, 116
Prostacyclin (PGI$_2$), 30, 31
Prostaglandins (PG), 7, 9, 11, 12–14, 23, 34, 43, 91, 92–93
Protein kinase C, 105
Prothrombin time (PT), 118
Psoriasis, 90–91
Pyrexia. *See* Fever.

Restenosis, 65–66
Reye's syndrome, 23
Rofecoxib. *See* Vioxx.

Schizophrenia, 101–102
Sears, Barry, 46, 113
Sed rate test, 16
Signal transduction, 101
Simopoulos, Artemis P., 41
Sinclair, Hugh, 61
Sjögren's syndrome, 89
Soy, 76
Statins, 66, 114
Steroids, 20–21, 32, 83
Stomach, 22
Strokes, 21, 27, 28, 76–78
Sulfites, 86
Synovium, 80

Systematic lupus erythematosus (SLE), 84–85

T lymphocytes, 69–70
Tears, 88
Third-party verification, 108
Thrombosis, 74
Thromboxane A$_2$, 32
Thromboxanes (TX), 9, 11, 14, 21, 30, 31, 34, 43
TNF-alpha, 46
Tofu, 76
Totox value, 112
Toxins, 16, 41, 50, 51
Triglycerides, 34, 66, 71, 74–75, 76, 109, 114–115
Tufts Report. *See Effects of Omega-3 Fatty Acids on Cardiovascular Risk Factors and Intermediate Markers of Cardiovascular Disease.*
Tufts University, 72

U.S. Food and Drug Administration (FDA), 18–19, 38, 56, 91
Ulcers, 14, 20, 22

Valdecoxib. *See* Bextra.
Vane, John, 23
Vascular disease, 58, 60, 67–72
Vasodilation, 71
Vein graft occlusion, 64
VIGOR (Vioxx Gastrointestinal Outcomes Research), 27, 104
Vioxx, 2, 14, 24, 27–29, 30, 60
Vitamin A, 108, 119
Vitamin D, 108, 119
Vitamin E, 111–112, 119

Walnuts, 14, 50, 76
Warfarin (Coumadin), 118–119

Zone, The (Sears), 46, 113

About the Authors

How does Dr. **Joseph C. Maroon,** a world-renowned neurosurgeon, team neurosurgeon for the Pittsburgh Steelers, and expert and international authority on concussion, orbital and brain tumors, minimally invasive surgery of the spine, and many neurosurgical diseases, become a proponent of fish oil? It truly has been a long, strange journey, but in many ways it has been a natural path based on Dr. Maroon's education, family background, natural passion for sports and health, and lifetime's work helping others.

Dr. Maroon was born in the upper Ohio valley, which encompasses northern West Virginia, southeastern Ohio, and southwestern Pennsylvania. His family was of modest means, and his father had a very strong influence on him, encouraging him to develop a strong work ethic and a desire to achieve, compete, and win. These qualities, along with a natural gift for both athletics and academics, helped him excel both on the playing field and in the classroom; he was his high-school class salutatorian, and he was awarded a football scholarship to Indiana University, where he was an academic All-American. He went on to medical school at IU and trained in neurosurgery at a number of prestigious hospitals and universities, including Georgetown University, the University of Vermont, and Oxford University in England. His professional career has since been marked with success, including appointment as a university chairman of the department of neurosurgery and surgery and as president of the Congress of Neurological Surgeons.

Dr. Maroon's life, however, changed dramatically after the death of his father at the age of sixty of a myocardial infarction. At this time, at the peak of his professional career, Dr. Maroon was faced with the realization that his family health history leaned heavily toward cardiac and cerebrovascular disease. This life-changing event led him to pursue significant preventive measures in his lifestyle to avoid what was considered an inevitable occurrence in the Maroon family: heart disease. He turned to running, which both helped relieve the stress of being a neurosurgeon and began to have significant health benefits. His blood pressure normalized, the amount of body fat he carried decreased, and his muscle tone and stamina improved. He was better able to focus on his work and was not completely exhausted, as he had been in the past, after long hours of surgery. He also began a quest to eat healthy foods and to explore dietary supplements and vitamins.

This was in the late 1970s and early 1980s, when the idea of exercise and the use of supplements to improve health was still considered a fringe theory and certainly not a mainstream idea. Dr. Maroon was unable to find much scientific information on what was the best exercise regime, what types of supplements to take to prevent disease, and more important, what nonpharmaceutical treatments were available to help prevent disease and especially heart disease. Having a personal stake in the prevention of premature cardiac death prompted him to attend many seminars on preventive health care and fitness. This journey often brought him to the arenas of nontraditional medicine, because the established medical system he had been a part of generally ignored or refused to believe anything outside of what was taught in medical school.

Dr. Maroon eventually became an expert in fitness and nutrition. His medical colleagues turned to him for information on preventive medicine and dietary supplements. He began to give his patients, who often were better informed about these topics than their physicians, information and personalized recommendations on exercise, diet, and supplements to improve their medical conditions. As team neurosurgeon to the Pittsburgh Steelers and neurosurgical consultant to many high-profile athletes, he began to provide information on appropriate supplements to help athletes with their chronic injuries and joint pain and inflammation. And he put into practice what he preaches by becoming a world-class triathlete, participating in World Ironman Triathlon Championships (2.5-mile swim, 125-mile bike, and 26-mile run) in Hawaii (twice), Canada, New Zealand, and Germany.

After more than twenty years as a practicing neurosurgeon and athlete, Dr. Maroon himself began to have joint pain and stiffness and, like most people, would either buy and take an over-the-counter nonsteroidal anti-inflammatory (NSAID), like Motrin or Aleve, or ask his doctor for a prescription for a more powerful NSAID like Vioxx, Celebrex, or Bextra. These pharmaceuticals gave him good relief, and he was able to continue his sport. However, his use of these NSAIDs came to an immediate halt after he attended a complementary medicine/anti-aging conference in 2002, at which time he learned of the serious side effects he had been exposing his patients and himself to while taking these NSAIDs. Annually, more than 100,000 hospitalizations and 16,000 deaths from gastric side effects and bleeding ulcers are associated with taking NSAIDs. More recently, with the Merck Company's withdrawal of Vioxx from the market, we have learned of the serious risk of heart attack and stroke carried by these widely promoted, widely prescribed, but dangerous drugs.

At this same conference Dr. Maroon learned of the scientific data on omega-3 essential fatty acids, which are found in fish oil, and how their mechanism of action, among many other functions, is to act as a natural anti-inflammatory. Having tried it on himself with great effectiveness, he began recommending fish oil to his patients as a natural alternative treatment for joint pain and stiffness and for the many other ailments noted in this book. He soon became a firm believer in the efficacy of fish oil as an anti-inflammatory treatment that doesn't involve the serious side effects of prescription drugs.

Dr. Maroon has since become one of the nation's leading advocates of fish oil and has lectured on the topic at major medical meetings nationally. His desire to spread the word about fish oil and its miraculous preventive and health-improving qualities has led to the drafting of this book. This book is dedicated to furthering our knowledge about the health benefits of fish oil and is intended to serve as a reference and education tool for both health professionals and the general public.

Jeffrey Bost, P.A.C., is a physician's assistant and clinical instructor in neuro-surgery. He has worked with Dr. Maroon for nearly twenty years in the operating room, in patient care, and as a scientific research coordinator and writer. Mr. Bost shares the same passion as Dr. Maroon for healthy living and sound nutrition and has published numerous articles with Dr. Maroon on both neurosurgical and nutritional subjects.